NUCLEAR CARDIOLOGY FOR CLINICIANS

Edited by

Jagmeet Singh Soin, M.D., F.A.C.C.
Associate Professor of Radiology and Medicine
Director, Nuclear Cardiology Laboratories
The Medical College of Wisconsin
Milwaukee County Medical Complex
Milwaukee, Wisconsin

and

Harold L. Brooks, M.D., F.A.C.C.
Professor of Medicine and Pharmacology
Chief, Cardiology Division
The Medical College of Wisconsin
Milwaukee, Wisconsin

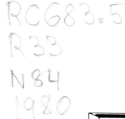

FUTURA PUBLISHING COMPANY
Mount Kisco, New York
1980

Dedication

This book is dedicated to our wives, Prabjot Kaur Soin and Carolyn Brooks.

Copyright © 1980
Futura Publishing Company, Inc.

Published by
Futura Publishing Company, Inc.
P.O. Box 330, 295 Main Street
Mount Kisco, New York 10549

LC #: 79-66870
ISBN #: 0-87993-131-0

Contributors

Masood Ahmad, M.D.
Assistant Professor of Medicine; Director, Non-invasive Cardiology Laboratory, University of Missouri Medical Center, Columbia, Missouri

Philip O. Alderson, M.D.
Associate Professor of Radiology; Associate Director of Nuclear Medicine, The Johns Hopkins Medical Institutions, Baltimore, Maryland

Virinderjit S. Bamrah, M.D.
Associate Professor of Medicine, The Medical College of Wisconsin, Milwaukee, Wisconsin; Assistant Chief, Cardiovascular Section and Director, Cardiac Catheterization Laboratory, Veterans Administration Hospital, Wood, Wisconsin

John Bingham, M.D.
Fellow in Nuclear Medicine, Massachusetts General Hospital, Boston, Massachusetts

Frederick J. Bonte, M.D.
Professor of Radiology; Dean, Southwestern Medical School, The University of Texas Health Sciences Center at Dallas, Dallas, Texas

Thomas J. Brady, M.D.
Fellow, Division of Nuclear Medicine, The University of Michigan Medical Center, Ann Arbor, Michigan

Harold L. Brooks, M.D.
Professor of Medicine and Pharmacology; Chief, Division of Cardiology, The Medical College of Wisconsin, Milwaukee, Wisconsin

L. Maximillian Buja, M.D.
Associate Professor of Pathology, Southwestern Medical School, The University of Texas Health Sciences Center at Dallas, Dallas, Texas

James E. Carey, M.S.
Assistant Professor of Radiation Physics, Departments of Radiology and Internal Medicine, The University of Michigan Medical Center, Ann Arbor, Michigan

Michael A. Davis, D.Sc.
Associate Professor of Radiology; Director, Joint Program in Nuclear Medicine Radiopharmacy, Harvard Medical School, Boston, Massachusetts

Richard Gorlin, M.D.
Murray M. Rosenberg Professor of Medicine; Chairman, Department of Medicine, Mount Sinai Medical Center, New York, New York

Charles M. Gross, M.D.
Assistant Professor of Medicine, Division of Cardiology, The Medical College of Wisconsin, Milwaukee, Wisconsin

Timothy E. Guiney, M.D.
Clinical Instructor in Medicine, Assistant Physician, Massachusetts General Hospital, Boston, Massachusetts

Robert E. Henkin, M.D.
Associate Professor of Radiology, Loyola University Medical Center; Director, Division of Nuclear Medicine, Foster G. McGaw Hospital, Maywood, Illinois

B. Leonard Holman, M.D.
Associate Professor of Radiology, Harvard Medical School; Chief, Clinical Nuclear Medicine, Peter Bent Brigham Hospital, Boston, Massachusetts

Michael H. Keelan, Jr., M.D.
Professor of Medicine, Division of Cardiology, The Medical College of Wisconsin, Milwaukee, Wisconsin

Samuel E. Lewis, M.D.
Assistant Professor of Radiology, Southwestern Medical School; Director, Division of Nuclear Medicine, The University of Texas Health Sciences Center at Dallas, Dallas, Texas

Randolph P. Martin, M.D.
Assistant Professor of Medicine; Director, Non-invasive Cardiology Laboratory, The University of Virginia School of Medicine, Charlottesville, Virginia

Kenneth A. McKusick, M.D.
Assistant Professor of Radiology, Harvard Medical School; Associate Radiologist, Massachusetts General Hospital; Clinical Director, Division of Nuclear Medicine, Massachusetts General Hospital, Boston, Massachusetts

Robert W. Parkey, M.D.
Professor and Chairman, Department of Radiology, Southwestern Medical School, The University of Texas Health Sciences Center at Dallas, Dallas, Texas

Bertram Pitt, M.D.

Professor of Internal Medicine; Chief, Division of Cardiology, The University of Michigan Medical Center, Ann Arbor, Michigan

Gerald M. Pohost, M.D.

Assistant Professor of Medicine, Massachusetts General Hospital, Boston, Massachusetts

Michael E. Siegel, M.D.

Associate Professor of Radiology, The University of Southern California School of Medicine; Radiologist, LAC/USC Medical Center, Los Angeles, California

Jagmeet S. Soin, M.D.

Director, Nuclear Cardiology Laboratories, and Associate Professor of Radiology and Medicine, The Medical College of Wisconsin, Milwaukee, Wisconsin; Clinical Professor, The University of Wisconsin-LaCrosse, LaCrosse, Wisconsin

Charles A. Stewart, M.D.

Fellow, Division of Nuclear Medicine, LAC/USC Medical Center, Los Angeles, California

H. William Strauss, M.D.

Associate Professor of Radiology, Harvard Medical School; Director, Division of Nuclear Medicine, Massachusetts General Hospital, Boston, Massachusetts

James H. Thrall, M.D.

Associate Professor of Internal Medicine and Radiology; Director, Division of Nuclear Cardiology, The University of Michigan Medical Center, Ann Arbor, Michigan

Donald D. Tresch, M.D.

Associate Professor of Medicine, Division of Cardiology, The Medical College of Wisconsin, Milwaukee, Wisconsin

Ramesh C. Verma, M.D.

Assistant Professor in Radiological Sciences (Nuclear Medicine Division), The University of California School of Medicine, Los Angeles; Director, Nuclear Medicine Division, Los Angeles County-UCLA Olive View Medical Center, Van Nuys, California

Henry N. Wagner, Jr., M.D.

Professor of Radiology, Medicine and Environmental Health Sciences; Director, Divisions of Nuclear Medicine and Radiation Health, The Johns Hopkins Medical Institutions, Baltimore, Maryland

Lee Samuel Wann, M.D.
Assistant Professor of Medicine; Director, Echocardiography, The Medical College of Wisconsin, Milwaukee, Wisconsin

James T. Willerson, M.D.
Professor of Internal Medicine, Southwestern Medical School; Director, Ischemic Heart Center, The University of Texas Health Sciences Center at Dallas, Dallas, Texas

James E. Youker, M.D.
Professor and Chairman, Department of Radiology, The Medical College of Wisconsin, Milwaukee, Wisconsin

Foreword

Nuclear medicine has been used primarily to obtain static images of vital organs. The application of this modality to cardiac diagnosis, however, takes advantage of nuclear medicine's unique ability to demonstrate function as well as anatomy. An accurate, noninvasive method of evaluating cardiac disorders has enormous potential in view of the high incidence of heart disease in our population.

This text is designed to explain the complexities of cardiac nuclear medicine to the practicing physician who encounters heart disease daily in his practice. This rapidly changing, highly technical field is confusing even to the experts, let alone to the clinician trying to decide which new diagnostic technique will be best for his patient.

Dr. Soin and Dr. Brooks have assembled contributions from an outstanding group of co-authors. The highly controversial issues of nuclear cardiac imaging are faced squarely. This text promises to be of inestimable value to the practicing physician.

James E. Youker

Preface

Cardiovascular disorders represent one of the greatest challenges facing the modern day clinician. The spectacular therapeutic advances made in the management of many acquired and congenital cardiac abnormalities have brought mounting pressures upon the clinician to provide the benefit of such advanced treatment to as many patients as possible. To add to his dilemma there are bewildering numbers of new diagnostic procedures which continually test his conventional diagnostic ability. Undoubtedly, cardiac catheterization, which allows the study of abnormal cardiac anatomy and physiology as well as the hemodynamic consequences, remains the "gold standard", and the newer noninvasive tests should supplement or complement this invasive study. In addition, the noninvasive tests not only should fit into the diagnostic evaluation of the patient, but also enable the physician to achieve the once elusive objectives of early detection of cardiac disease and possible prevention.

Cardiovascular applications of radionuclides are not new to the diagnostic field, but it is only recently that sufficient experience and technical sophistication have been achieved so that these techniques can be utilized optimally in routine evaluation of cardiac patients.

The purpose of writing this book is to present in a basic and simple form the tremendous advances made in noninvasive evaluation of a cardiac patient, and also to illustrate the ease with which the effects of various cardiac disorders on cardiac function can now be evaluated. In this book we have attempted to point out the relative merits of radionuclide studies in evaluation of a cyanotic child suspected of having congenital heart disease, as well as an adult suffering from peripheral vascular disease. We do not intend to offer this book as a comprehensive textbook of cardiovascular nuclear medicine, but rather a composite critique of several radionuclide studies which have proved to be simple, reproducible, specific, sensitive and easily applicable within a clinical nuclear medicine laboratory.

This book primarily focuses on the needs of the community hospitals which are considering the possibility of starting a noninvasive cardiac diagnostic facility. In this day and age of cost-effectiveness, optimal utilization of any given equipment is of paramount importance. A critical appraisal of equipment needs, data processing units and portable gamma scintillation cameras will be made in some detail to justify their purchase based on practical applications. Finally, we hope that this book will help in developing a working knowledge in this field and allow the reader to use these new diagnostic modalities as an adjunct to cardiac catheterization in some instances, and where appropriate, as a reasonable alternative. Radionuclide studies can, when properly used, provide the necessary information for accurate follow-up after therapeutic interventions.

We have purposely excluded any discussion of elaborate nuclear medicine techniques such as microsphere perfusion or xenon washout studies of coronary circulation. Interested readers can use standard textbooks on these subjects. Also omitted from consideration are the techniques of the future, such as positron cameras and positron emitting radiopharmaceuticals. Guest authors have been carefully selected from the leaders in this specialty in the United States. We acknowledge their contributions in preparation of this book with deep gratitude.

It was readily understood by us that any new book on cardiovascular nuclear medicine faces the dangers of becoming obsolete in a comparatively short time; however, if it addresses the fundamental question, "How can these new techniques be understood by more clinicians in the community hospitals?" the chances of acceptance of such a textbook become quite high. It is to fulfill this objective that the contributors have devoted their time and efforts. Any task of this magnitude also puts the entire team through a rigorous drill. Needless to mention, without the untiring efforts of Mrs. Susan E. Gavran in assisting with library work and typing, and the editorial assistance of Mrs. Dianna Stearman Lawrence, the accomplishment of this objective would have remained an unfulfilled dream. We wish to give special thanks to David W. Palmer, Ph.D. and Mrs. Lorie Pelc for reviewing key manuscripts. We would be remiss not to offer our appreciation to all the laboratory personnel who hesitantly learned to cope with "withdrawn bosses" in both the nuclear medicine and cardiology divisions. We hope that this book will narrow the gap between advances taking place in academic centers and the community hospitals in this important new area of nuclear cardiology.

Jagmeet S. Soin
Harold L. Brooks

Contents

CHAPTER I

Introduction to Cardiovascular Nuclear Medicine

Henry N. Wagner, Jr., M.D.

Progress in medicine has followed advances in our perception of bodily structure and function as well as in our concept of disease processes. In 1806 with the publication of Corvisart's book "Diseases of the Heart," "observation" of patients became "examination". Corvisart describes pericarditis, dilation and hypertrophy of the heart, and diseases of the heart muscle, valves and aorta. His use of percussion allowed him to surpass all his predecessors in clinical skills, and his book is full of excellent case histories and autopsy correlations. He propagated Auenbrugger's invention until by 1825, it was used generally in Paris and had spread everywhere from there. With the use of percussion, medicine became less "conjectural". Corvisart was the inventor of the heart function test. His student René Laennec invented the stethoscope and then described it in his 1819 "Treatise on Mediate Ausculation and on the Diseases of the Lung and Heart." Together, ausculation and percussion made possible a kind of living pathological anatomy or anatomical pathology.

Einthoven developed the string galvanometer to record the electrical changes accompanying each heart beat. Soon, Sir Thomas Lewis began to use the instrument in England and to correlate resulting data with clinical observations. Today, the electrocardiogram is an indispensible aid to modern cardiologists. Electrocardiography and with it, modern cardiology, evolved from Einthoven's original development. The next major technical advance was the development of cardiac catheterization and contrast angiography, both essential to the growth of modern cardiovascular surgery.

Adapted from Lewis A. Conner Memorial Lecture, 51st Annual Meeting of the American Heart Association, Dallas, Texas.

Few persons realize that the first diagnostic uses of radioactive tracers were not in the study of the thyroid, but in the study of the heart. Blumgart and Weiss saw the potential of radioactive tracers in diagnosis and began their studies only a few years after Einthoven won the Nobel Prize. In 1927 they described their studies of normal persons and patients with heart disease. When we think about their use of radium salt solution as a tracer and a cloud chamber as a detector, we can appreciate the enormous advances made over the last half century. The prospect of using radioactive tracers to study the heart has now become a reality with the invention of suitable instruments and radioactive tracers.

The growth of the field of nuclear cardiology over the past few years can be seen in Figure 1-1 which shows the increase in number of the two most common nuclear cardiology studies performed today in the John Hopkins Hospital, the thallium-201 myocardial perfusion study and the

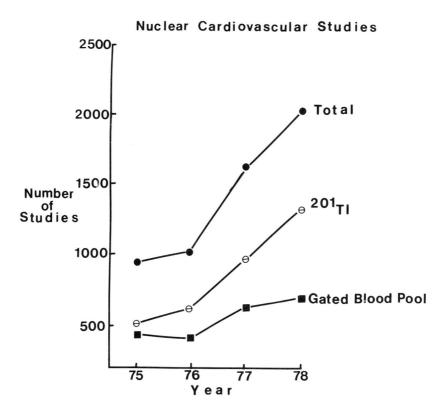

Figure. 1-1.   Nuclear cardiovascular studies performed at the Johns Hopkins Hospital during the years 1975-78.

ventricular function test. Initially these studies were used primarily in the diagnosis of the cause of chest pain. They are also used in the differential diagnosis of patients with dyspnea, in patients with unexplained heart murmurs, and in children with cyanosis.

Measurements that can now be made with intravenous injection of radioactive tracers include:

1. Right and left ventricular volumes
2. Right and left ventricular hypertrophy
3. Cardiac output at rest and exercise
4. Mitral and aortic valvular regurgitation
5. Right-to-left and left-to-right shunt quantification
6. Global and regional wall motion of the right and left ventricle
7. Regional myocardial blood flow
8. Left ventricular work and power

It will take years of further research to refine these measurements and define their precision, accuracy, indications and utility, but even today we can conclude that they will probably continue to play a major role in clinical cardiology and cardiovascular research. For example, among the questions now being asked of these studies are the following:

1. What is the cause of the patient's chest pain?
2. What is the hemodynamic significance of electrocardiographic abnormalities such as premature ventricular beats and atrial fibrillation?
3. Has the patient had myocardial infarction?
4. How much of the left ventricular muscle is involved?
5. How recent is the infarction?
6. What is the patient's right and left ventricular function at rest, during exercise, or after drugs?
7. Does the patient have a ventricular aneurysm?
8. Does the patient have a complication of infarction such as mitral regurgitation or a ruptured septum?
9. Is the right ventricle affected by infarction?
10. Does the patient have transient ischemia in addition to fixed perfusion defects at rest?

In patients with dyspnea, the questions being asked include:

1. Does the patient have predominantly lung disease with normal cardiac function?
2. What is the relative involvement of perfusion and ventilation?

3. Does the patient have cor pulmonale as evidenced by right ventricular ejection fraction?
4. What is the relative involvement of the right ventricle, lungs and left ventricle?

Although nuclear cardiology has been used for nearly a decade in the diagnosis of congenital heart disease, for example in differentiating cardiac from non-cardiac causes of cyanosis, the use of these studies has not increased as dramatically as the use of those used to evaluate coronary heart disease. Echocardiography has become the screening procedure of choice in these patients. Nevertheless, in detection of intracardiac shunts and complicated congenital diseases, the tracer studies are probably the most sensitive and accurate methods to quantitate left-to-right shunts.

Of course, the nuclear studies will never replace cardiac catheterization and contrast angiography. This is seen clearly in Figure 1-2 which shows the concomitant increase in patients studied by cardiac catheterization at Johns Hopkins Hospital during the period of rapid growth of the nuclear studies (and echocardiography). Since each of the modalities—history, physical examination, electrocardiography, echocardiography, nuclear cardiology, cardiac catheterization and contrast angiocardiography—provides a different type of information, that is, each assesses something different, it seems unlikely that one will replace the other. For many patients the noninvasive tests will replace the invasive studies. For example, it is no longer necessary to perform coronary angiography to exclude a diagnosis of coronary heart disease with 90 percent certainty in an airline pilot who had an abnormal electrocardiogram on routine examination; or to perform ventriculography to exclude aneurysm in patients with demonstrably diffuse hypokinesis. Noninvasive testing is also being used in patients for whom invasive studies are not thought justified as a screening test. At times the noninvasive techniques reveal abnormalities at early stages when corrective measures can still reverse or arrest the disease process. Assessment of ventricular function in patients with left-to-right shunts is an example of such a use. Another example is the finding of abnormal ventricular function in patients with hypothyroidism. Finally, in patients with noncoronary cardiomyopathies, such as sarcoidosis, involvement of the myocardium can be diagnosed early by noninvasive techniques.

Much of the research in nuclear cardiology today is concerned with trying to answer these questions:

1. What are the relative advantages and disadvantages of the various nuclear cardiology procedures, e.g., thallium-

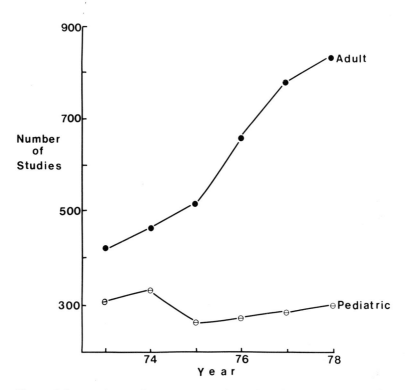

Figure 1-2.   Cardiac catheterizations performed at the Johns Hopkins Hospital.

201 imaging of regional myocardial perfusion and technetium-99m albumin or red blood cell imaging of ventricular function?

2. When should first transit of ECG-synchronized studies be performed?

3. Which is more accurate in the detection of coronary artery disease, thallium-201 exercise studies or gated blood pool studies during exercise?

4. Will the Anger camera remain the predominant imaging device?

5. How quantitive can the results be?

6. Will tomography improve detection of lesions such as subendocardial infarction where sensitivity today is still troublesome?

7. Can the 10 to 20 percent false negative rate for thallium-

201 exercise tests be decreased?
8. Will simpler special purpose devices become widespread, for example, in monitoring patients in conjunction with electrocardiography?
9. Will Swan-Ganz monitoring be replaced by ventricular function monitoring?

As recently as 40 years ago assessment of left ventricular function was limited to the appearance of congestion or shock. Subsequently, methods were developed for cardiac diagnosis that clearly showed that clinical signs are insensitive and that dysfunctional changes precede clinical signs. The invention and application of nuclear and echocardiographic methods have allowed measurement of regional as well as global function. As with other organs, regional changes in the heart are often found before overall function falls outside the wide range of normal global function. This has been called the "homogeneity principle" and provides the basis for early diagnosis. The function of one part of the heart is compared to that of other parts, as in measurement of ventricular wall motion or the distribution of myocardial blood flow.

In addition to their usefulness in the differential diagnosis of chest pain, dyspnea and fatigue, nuclear methods can also serve in prognosis and planning treatment. For example, severely impaired left ventricular function can pose a relative contraindication to valvular or coronary artery surgery, while early ventricular failure may indicate the need for cardiac surgery in patients with intracardiac shunts. Drugs, such as propranolol or adriamycin, can be used more effectively if their effect on ventricular function can be monitored.

Perhaps the greatest appeal of nuclear cardiology is the visual display of function. Human beings derive nearly all their sensory input through their eyes. People are better at perception than conception, and therefore nuclear and echocardiographic images, especially when they are displayed as motion pictures are very convincing. The greatest limitation of the nuclear studies at the present time is quantification, although this is improving.

The radiation dose is low and decades of experience with exposures at the level of nuclear cardiology studies have not revealed any deleterious effects. The quality of today's images has improved greatly over the first lung scans or myocardial perfusion studies performed with potassium-43. Computers are now commonplace and are considered necessary for first-class cardiovascular nuclear medicine studies. Cinematic display on color television is now widely used. New collimators are being introduced. Tomography is providing important improvements in sensitivity and quantification. Sixteen new tomographic systems were reported at the last Society of Nuclear Medicine meeting, together with four special purpose systems that are much simpler than scintillation camera systems. At present, spatial resolution in imaging systems is limited to about 2 cubic centimeters with a precision of about 90 percent in quantitative assays done with tomography. It is likely that this figure will improve. Problems remain, but the future is bright.

In summary, the knowledge now being accumulated on radionuclide cardiovascular procedures has direct application to the care of cardiac patients. This book should help a reader to decide which procedures are best suited to help his or her patients.

CHAPTER II

Evaluation of the Cardiac Patient with Nuclear Techniques: An Overview

Harold L. Brooks, M.D., and Jagmeet S. Soin, M.D.

In the late 1960's a revolution in cardiology began with the application of noninvasive techniques in the diagnosis of heart disease. Advances in technology in two major areas, radionuclide imaging and echocardiography, essentially have provided the basis for this revolution. During the past decade, imaging of the heart and circulatory system using radionuclides has markedly enhanced the practicing physician's capability for accurate and informative cardiac evaluation.[1]

While radioisotopes have been used in experimental medicine for many years, it is only recently that they have gained acceptance as legitimate diagnostic tests for the evaluation of common cardiopulmonary disorders. The diagnostic evaluation for pulmonary embolism, for example, is much different than it was just a decade ago, thanks to the availability of perfusion lung scans. The initial evaluation and follow-up of many patients with acute myocardial infarction and angina pectoris is changing because of the direct application of newfound capabilities of nuclear cardiac techniques to the day-to-day management of a cardiac patient. Three advances have made the progress in nuclear cardiology possible. The first is the development of gamma scintillation cameras with better spatial resolution, and improved collimators. The second is the availability of medically suitable radiopharmaceuticals which will selectively localize in the normal or damaged myocardial tissue. The third involves minicomputers and microprocessors which are now fast, powerful, and compact and allow the processing and storing of the characteristically large volumes of data at a relatively low cost. The detailed consideration of these principal factors has been provided in subsequent chapters in this book.

In cardiology and medicine, we have come to realize the usefulness of radionuclides as screening procedures to exclude heart disease, to determine the extent of the disease and follow its course, for the periodic examination in the asymptomatic patient, and in the assessment and follow-up of hemodynamic responses to newly developed cardiac rehabilitation programs. Radionuclide imaging in conjunction with coronary arteriography promises to have wide application in the initial evaluation and long-term follow-up of patients who have had acute myocardial infarction. By performing both invasive and noninvasive studies during the initial examination, specific relationships can be established between the two, and hence in many, extensive follow-up can be performed by noninvasive radionuclide studies exclusively. Radionuclide imaging has already proven valuable in quantitative assessment of the patient's hemodynamic and functional responses following coronary bypass surgery.

Radionuclide imaging techniques offer a real promise to the physician wanting a more precise quantitative assessment of the effect of therapeutic modalities upon the patient's cardiac function. Until recently, the primary diagnostic tool for the practicing physician was cardiac catheterization and angiography, which supplemented the clinical judgment based upon signs and symptomatology. Now, radionuclide techniques offer a fairly precise way to document and assess global and regional cardiac function and myocardial perfusion by relatively innocuous and comparatively inexpensive outpatient techniques.

Common Procedures in Nuclear Cardiology

The major nuclear medicine procedures for cardiac imaging of importance to the practicing physician fall into four categories: (1) radionuclide angiocardiogram, (2) myocardial perfusion scan, (3) myocardial infarct scanning and (4) gated blood pool study. The indications and use for these are summarized in Table 2-1.

Radionuclide Angiocardiogram

In this technique, a bolus of radionuclide tracer is injected intravenously and its subsequent passage is monitored as it passes through the central circulation and chambers of the heart using a nuclear detector, primarily a gamma scintillation camera. The primary use of this technique is in the evaluation of pediatric patients with suspected congenital heart disease.[2] This procedure is extremely safe and relatively

TABLE 2-1
Common Nuclear Cardiology Procedures

PROCEDURE	APPLICATION
1. RADIONUCLIDE ANGIOCARDIOGRAM	Detection of intracardiac shunts, screening for heart disease in infants, differentiating acute mitral regurgitation from ventricular septal defects in patients with acute myocardial infarction.
2. MYOCARDIAL PERFUSION SCAN	
Stress:	To detect regions of ischemia and scar.
Rest:	To detect regions of scar and acute infarction.
3. SCANNING WITH INFARCT AVID AGENTS	Detection of acute myocardial infarction.
4. GATED CARDIAC BLOOD POOL SCAN	Evaluation of left ventricular function, separation of localized from diffuse contraction abnormalities and aneurysm.

simple. The attendant radiation exposure is also comparatively low and is generally equal to the radiation dose given to the patient from a single chest radiograph. Its other major application is to determine whether cardiac catheterization should be performed in a child with heart murmur of undetermined origin. The radionuclide angiocardiogram can be quite useful in differentiating between hemodynamically insignificant murmurs, i.e., the functional murmurs, and murmurs requiring evaluation by cardiac catheterization such as those resulting from congenital cardiac abnormalities. Additionally, in each type of congenital heart disease, bolus transit through the central circulatory system is altered according to a certain recognizable pattern. This procedure can also be useful in differentiating between primary pulmonary disorders and congenital heart defects in neonates. Perhaps the most important aspect of radionuclide angiocardiography is in its ability not only to delineate the structural defect, but also to express it in a quantitative or semiquantitative manner through the use of relatively simple analytical methods.[3] Alderson describes these in detail in Chapter 18 of this book.

Myocardial Perfusion Imaging

Currently, primary clinical application of myocardial perfusion imaging is in the detection and localization of regional myocardial ischemia and infarction. There are two different approaches taken to assess the regional myocardial perfusion; one is invasive and the other is more simple and relatively noninvasive. The invasive method involves the selective injection of radiolabeled albumin microspheres or microaggregates directly into the coronary arteries during cardiac catheterization.[4] While the resultant images provide excellent information concerning regional myocardial perfusion, there remain many unresolved theoretic problems. Since this method requires cardiac catheterization, only a few laboratories are currently using this procedure, mostly on an experimental basis. It is our belief that this procedure has limited applications for the practicing physician. We shall limit further discussion of this important subject to the two major noninvasive methods which are currently in use at most clinics and hospitals.

Radionuclide Studies Dependent on Regional Myocardial Blood Flow

Earlier experience with potassium-43, rubidium-81, and ammonia N-13 has given way to the more popular thallium-201, with its more suitable physical characteristics.[5] The thallium perfusion scan is now widely used to evaluate patients with coronary artery disease and monitor the patient's response to therapy. The test is usually performed during, and several hours following exercise. The purpose of the exercise perfusion scan is to visualize regions of reduced myocardial perfusion which may be related to recent or old myocardial infarction, or to detect regions of the myocardium that are viable but become transiently ischemic during a stress state.[6] This test is helpful in selecting patients for coronary arteriography and possible surgery and as a means for monitoring the results of coronary bypass surgery. Under conditions of physical stress, the myocardial blood flow can increase two to three times in normal subjects. However, there is little increase in blood flow to the area supplied by coronary vessels with high grade fixed obstructions. The technique itself has had wide acceptance and has been reported to be more sensitive and specific for ischemic heart disease than other available techniques. Further detailed consideration of this subject is made in Chapters 3 and 5 through 9.

Radionuclides With Special Affinity for Acutely Infarcted Myocardium

The radiopharmaceuticals used to detect acute myocardial infarction include several technetium (^{99m}Tc) labeled compounds. The most notable among these are technetium-labeled phosphates, tetracycline and glucoheptonate. The most extensive clinical experience to date has been obtained with technetium stannous pyrophosphate.[7] Although the cellular basis for the avidity of these agents to the infarcted tissue is not clearly understood, it appears that they localize in a crystalline structure within the mitochondria of necrotic myocardial cells and then are incorporated into the hydroxyapatite crystals.[8] Clinically, the evidence of positive accumulation in infarcted myocardial tissue is seen within 12 to 18 hours after the onset of symptoms. The accumulation of radioactivity becomes more intense over the subsequent days for a period of two weeks. Parkey et al. in Chapter 10 and Ahmad in Chapter 12 discuss this technique, its uses and limitations further.

Gated Blood Pool Studies

Left ventricular function and regional wall motion can be analyzed with sequential gated scintillation images. A radionuclide, usually technetium-99m labeled to human serum albumin, is administered intravenously and it remains in the blood pool for several hours. More recently, new techniques of in-vivo labeling of patient's red blood cells have been utilized to have better blood pool agents. The electronic gate is then used which is triggered by the ECG. This gate enables the gamma scintillation camera to take images during the present and predefined portion of the cardiac cycle. The two periods generally selected are end-systole and end-diastole. The images are recorded in multiple projections to allow visualization and localization of regional wall motion abnormalities. The outline of the left ventricle is examined either by manual tracing of the border with a light pen, or more recently by a computerized edge detection and analysis program. The end-diastolic and end-systolic volumes are measured and the ejection fraction is calculated using standard hemodynamic formulae. Superimposing the traced outline of the ventricles at end-systole and end-diastole permit an evaluation of regional myocardial contractility. These methods were initially adapted to nuclear cardiology applications by Strauss et al.,[9] and then have been shown in several recent studies to correlate well with single plane left ventriculography.

This technique can be adapted to analyze initial passage of the radionuclide through the ventricle within its "first pass" or it can be adapted to multiple gated acquisition techniques ("MUGA"). In the first pass study, relatively high counts are necessary to obtain sufficient data during the short time it takes the radionuclide to travel through the ventricles. In the MUGA study, counts can be accumulated over a longer period of time. Both procedures are also adaptable to analysis during exercise and compared to a similar study performed at rest. The two studies can then be used to compare changes in ventricular function and regional wall motion induced by relative ischemia. Other interventions such as nitroglycerin administration, atrial pacing, and induced premature ventricular contractions have been used with good success. Detailed consideration of these techniques will be discussed by Thrall and Pitt in their Chapters 13 and 14.

The clinicans of the 1980's will depend heavily upon nuclear cardiac techniques for the definitive diagnosis and management of patients with cardiac disease. The wider acceptance of these techniques will be based upon the fact that they are fairly simple, atraumatic and do not require hospitalization. They can be repeated easily and the clinician can gather more useful quantitative information with a degree of accuracy in many cases equal to that of catheterization studies. The response to surgery, medications, and cardiac rehabilitation programs can be assessed by nuclear imaging techniques. The time course and long-term adaptive processes of the ventricular myocardium to obstructive coronary artery disease will be studied with these techniques in a manner not previously possible and no doubt yield information to the clinician not previously available.

References

1. Strauss, H.W.: Cardiovascular nuclear medicine. A new look at an old problem. *Radiology* **121**:257-266, 1976.
2. Wesselhoeft, H., Hurley, P.J., Wagner, H.N., Jr., et al.: Nuclear angiocardiography in the diagnosis of congenital heart disease in infants. *Circulation* **45**:77-91, 1972.

3. Treves, S., Maltz, D.L., and Adelstein, S.J.: Intracardiac shunts. In James, A.E., Jr., Wagner, H.N., Jr., and Cooke, R.E. (Eds.): *Pediatric Nuclear Medicine.* Philadelphia, W.B. Saunders Co., 1974, pp. 231-246.
4. Cannon, P.J., Dell, R.B., and Dwyer, E.M., Jr.: Regional myocardial perfusion rates in patients with coronary artery disease. *J Clin Invest* 51:978-994, 1972.
5. Lebowitz, E., Green, M.W., Fairchild, R., et al.: Thallium-201 for medical use. *J Nucl Med* 16:151-155, 1975.
6. Pohost, G.M., Zir, L.M., Moore, R.H., et al.: Differentiation of transiently ischemic from infarcted myocardium by serial imaging after a single dose of Thallium-201. *Circulation* 55:294-302, 1977.
7. Bruno, F.P., Cobb, F.R., Rivas, F., et al.: Evaluation of ^{99m} technetium stannous pyrophosphate as an imaging agent in acute myocardial infarction. *Circulation* 54:71-78, 1976.
8. Buja, L.M., Parkey, R.W., Stokely, E.M., et al.: Pathophysiology of technetium-99m stannous pyrophosphate and thallium-201 scintigraphy of acute anterior myocardial infarcts in dogs. *J Clin Invest* 57:1508-1522, 1976.
9. Strauss, H.W., Zaret, B.L., Hurley, P.J., et al.: A scintiphotographic method for measuring left ventricular ejection fraction in man without cardiac catheterization. *Am J Cardiol* 28:575-580, 1971.

CHAPTER III

Radiopharmaceuticals in Cardiovascular Nuclear Medicine

Michael A. Davis, D.Sc., and B. Leonard Holman, M.D.

Radioactive tracers have been used for over 50 years to evaluate cardiac and circulatory disorders,[1] but only recently have clinically relevant techniques been refined to the point where they are routine and efficacious. The need for noninvasive methods of evaluating the heart has created a renewal of interest in nuclear medicine techniques. As in the past, it has been the combination of the physician asking clinically relevant questions, the physicist responding to these needs by designing and building the necessary instrumentation, and the chemist tailoring the radiotracer to meet the physiological and physical requirements of the human body, respectively, that has led to the development of new nuclear diagnostic procedures.

Basic Physical and Biological Considerations

In the discussion of any class of organ-specific radiopharmaceuticals, one must consider the properties of the radionuclide separately from those of the carrier molecule. Before describing the radiopharmaceuticals used in nuclear cardiology, a review of the physical properties of radionuclides and the criteria for their incorporation into carrier molecules is essential.

The decay scheme of a radionuclide is the most important consideration in determining its suitability for incorporation into a radiopharmaceutical. The term "decay scheme" encompasses such factors as type of radioactive emissions, energy of emitted rays, nature and stability of daughter(s) isotopes produced, and the physical half-life of both parent and daughter(s).

Nuclear Disintegration Processes

The nuclear disintegration processes are outlined in Table 3-1. In diagnostic nuclear medicine it is important to use radionuclides having a minimum of nonpenetrating radiation (beta or very low energy gamma radiation), since particles that do not escape from the body add no diagnostic information but significantly increase the absorbed radiation dose to the patient. For this reason, radionuclides which decay by isomeric transition and emit penetrating radiation, i.e., gamma rays, are preferred. The amount of internal conversion occurring is also important since the converted and Auger electrons along with low energy characteristic x-rays detract from photon emission and increase patient absorbed radiation dose. Therefore, they are undesirable for clinical use. Figure 3-1 shows the decay by isomeric transition for ^{99m}Tc, the most commonly used radioisotope. There are two routes by which this metastable state of technetium can decay: 0.68 percent of the 142 keV disintegrations go directly to the ground state (^{99}Tc) and are almost entirely converted; whereas, 99.32 percent of the decay goes from the 142 keV plateau to a 140 keV energy level by losing 2 keV by internal conversion. The 140 keV state decays to ground level with little internal conversion (116 conversion electrons/1000 photons; conversion coefficient α = .116). Thus, ^{99m}Tc can, for all practical purposes, be considered to emit a monoenergetic gamma ray of 140 keV with only a small amount of nonpenetrating radiation arising from Auger and conversion electrons.

Of the remaining nuclear disintegration processes shown in Table 3-1, there has been some success with two types of isobaric transition: positron decay and electron capture. Positrons have an energy spectrum similar in shape to the β-decay spectrum. They are detected as 511 keV photons arising as they collide with orbital electrons. The two oppositely charged particles are attracted to each other by electrical force and a product of their collision (annihilation) are two 511 keV photons that carry off the energy at paths 180° to each other. Relatively few positron-emitting nuclides have sufficiently long half-lives to be useful in nuclear medicine. Some that have found considerable utility are: sodium-22, fluorine-18, gallium-68, arsenic-74, copper-64, and more recently the cyclotron-produced gases containing carbon-11, nitrogen-13 and oxygen-15.

The second type of isobaric transition is electron capture. The end result of the electron capture decay process is the ejection of a single neutrino from the nucleus (itself of no practical use in radionuclide scanning) and emission of a series of electronic x-ray photons and Auger

TABLE 3-1.

Nuclear Disintegration Processes

Type	Symbol	Radiation Emitted	Change in Nucleus	
			Z^*	$A\dagger$
1. Isomeric Transitions				
Gamma-ray Decay	γ	Gamma-ray	0	0
Internal Conversion	e(I.C.)	Electron (e^-), characteristic x-rays, Auger electrons, bremsstrahlung photons	0	0
2. Isobaric Transitions				
Beta Decay	β^-	Electron, neutrino, bremsstrahlung	+1	0
Positron Decay	$\beta+$	Positron, neutrino, bremsstrahlung, annihilation photons	-1	0
Electron Capture	e.c.	Neutrino, characteristic x-rays, Auger electrons	-1	0
3. Alpha Decay	α	Alpha-ray	-2	-4

*Z = number of protons

†A = atomic mass

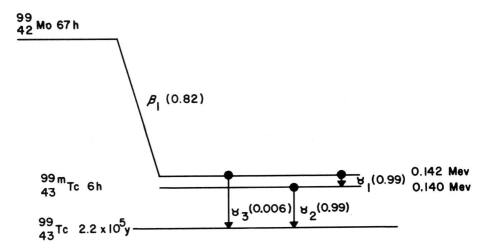

Figure 3-1.   Schematic representation of the decay scheme of technetium-99m.

electrons from the atom. In the past, with the exception of iodine-125, nuclides that decay by electron capture were seldom used. However, they are becoming increasingly popular because the radiation is almost entirely in the form of low energy photons and neutrinos with few high energy electrons; there is no beta or positron radiation, and the half-life is usually of reasonable duration. The two remaining types of decay (beta and alpha) have no use in diagnostic in vivo procedures, but have found application in in-vitro assays and in therapy.

Product of Radioactive Decay

The nuclide produced as the result of radioactive decay of another nuclide (referred to as the daughter and parent, respectively) also must be considered when evaluating a radionuclide's potential as a component of a radiopharmaceutical. In an ideal situation the daughter is stable (non-radioactive), or has an extremely long half-life so that when compared to the human life span it can be considered stable. As a parent, ^{99m}Tc falls into this category since its daughter, ^{99}Tc, has a half-life of 2×10^5 years.

Energy of Emitted Gamma Ray

Another important consideration in selecting a suitable radioisotope is its photon energy. The radiation detection system has two main components that influence the choice of photon energy, the collimator and the scintillation crystal. Collimators have been designed to provide either resolution or sensitivity at both low (80 to 200 keV) and moderate (300 to 500 keV) energy levels. From a practical standpoint, it becomes difficult to collimate photons accurately when they have energies in excess of 500 keV. Three- and five-inch diameter sodium iodide scintillation crystals used in rectilinear scanners are sufficiently sensitive and give resolution (with the appropriate collimator) up to 400 to 500 keV. However, the large diameter crystal used with scintillation cameras (11 in. diameter or greater) is thinner than the 3- and 5-inch scanning crystals and therefore not nearly as efficient in capturing higher energy photons. As a general rule, scanners are designed to operate at maximum efficiency in the 200 to 400 keV range, whereas the gamma cameras operate best in the 100 to 250 keV range.

Physical Half-life (T_p)

Theoretically, any radionuclide being considered for incorporation into a radiopharmaceutical should have the shortest physical half-life (T_p) compatible with the physiologic half-period of the phenomenon under study. Wagner has indicated that, based upon mathematical considerations, the ideal half-life of a radionuclide should be 0.693 times the length of time necessary to complete the diagnostic procedures (0.693 T).[2] The advantages of using short-lived radiopharmaceuticals are listed in Table 3-2. However, the definition of ideal half-life depends upon the type of study being performed (static versus dynamic) and the nature of the study (number of views, repeat views, etc.). For dynamic studies which may need to be repeated, isotopes with ultra-short half-lives would be preferable. Since most static studies take from 30 to 120 minutes, the optimal half-life for desirable radionuclides ranges from 4 hours to 3 days. Radionuclides having half-lives of less than 24 hours must be available in generator form to attain widespread acceptance, whereas nuclides having half-lives of 3 days can be supplied in "ready to inject" pharmaceutical form by commercial vendors. An example of the former is ^{99m}Tc (T_p = 6.1 hours), and of the latter, thallium-201 (T_p = 73 hours). The radionuclide gases are a notable exception to this rule because of their extremely short biological half-lives. In these situations the dose to the patient is minimal and the overriding considerations are shelflife and economics. A good example is xenon-133 which has a half-life of approximately 5 days.

TABLE 3-2

Advantages and Disadvantages of Short-Lived Radiopharmaceuticals*

ADVANTAGES

1. Reduced radiation exposure to patients.
2. Markedly reduced radioactive contamination hazard.
3. Increased photon yield. Leads to improve counting statistics and better resolution.
4. Allows additional studies (repeat or new) at frequent intervals without interference from the previously administered radiopharmaceutical.
5. Less time required to complete diagnostic procedure (more photons) permitting more patients to be examined.

DISADVANTAGES

1. Many agents require "on-site" preparation. Necessitates special facilities and personnel.
2. Production and quality control more difficult.
3. Potentially higher levels of radiation exposure to personnel during preparation.
4. Short shelf life after formulation. Often require multiple preparations daily.
5. Ultra short-lived nuclides decay substantially during the period of measurement. Decay correction must be applied.
6. Long-term follow-up of distribution or metabolism (24-, 48- or 72-hour studies) not possible.

*For this table the definition of short-lived is 8 hours or less.

Availability and Cost

The availability of radionuclides with long half-lives is no problem. Their long physical life allows their purchase either weekly or every other week. However, requirements for the high levels of short-lived radionuclides make a continuous supply more difficult and expensive. The availability of radionuclide generators has solved this problem.

From 1967 to 1971 nearly all the technetium used in hospital-based nuclear medicine clinics was eluted from ^{99}Mo-^{99m}Tc-radionuclide generators. Technetium-99m can also be separated from ^{99}Mo in quantity for distribution by extraction with organic solvents such as methyl-ethyl ketone. This separated ^{99m}Tc can be provided in a pharmaceutical grade, at any desired specific activity, while the parent ^{99}Mo is retained by the supplier. However, because of the relatively short half-life of ^{99m}Tc, the problems of quality control, scheduling, shipping and meeting daily requirements of the various technetium-labeled agents are great. Thus, the utility of these ready-to-use or so-called "instant" technetium products is limited to users located within a short distance of the supplier. Additionally, emergency needs on nights and weekends are a serious concern. On the other hand, the advantages of receiving the radiopharmaceutical precalibrated in a form ready for use, considered together with the overall economics, can make this method the best one for those located near a commercial supplier. Technetium pertechnetate $(^{99m}$TcO$_4^-)$ can be converted to other chemical forms much more easily by the supplier than by small hospitals lacking the proper facilities and personnel.

Biochemical Criteria

Biologic and Effective Half-life

The physical half-life of a radionuclide is only one of the factors involved in computing the radiation dose to the biological systems. The chemical form of a radionuclide will determine its biologic distribution. In living systems, each tissue or organ has its own way of eliminating materials, and this method of clearance must be considered when determining the residence time of a radiopharmaceutical in any organ. This biological removal can be expressed as the biological halftime (T_b) provided this agent clears the tissues exponentially. The biologic halftime is related to an excretion rate in the same manner that the physical half-life is related to a disintegration rate. If a radioactive compound is located in an organ, and that organ excretes the compound at a specific rate, then the radioactivity has an even greater rate of disappearance than would be expected, based solely on the rate of physical decay. This combined clearance rate has been designated as the effective clearance rate and is most often expressed numerically as the effective half-life (T_{eff}). Since the physical and biological half-life of any radioactive material can be measured experimentally, the effective half-life can be computed by solving the equation as shown:

$$T_{eff} = \frac{T_p \times T_b}{T_p + T_b}$$

The mechanisms involved in excreting radioactive material from living systems are often complex and not adequately described by simple exponential clearance curves. For accurate kinetic studies, biologic clearance can generally be expressed as linear sums of exponential values with constant coefficients. In these cases the term 50 percent clearance time or 50 percent retention time should be used, and the dose calculations should comprise as many 50 percent clearance values as are necessary to account for the total radiation exposure.

Keeping these fundamental considerations in mind, we will now describe the radiopharmaceuticals developed for clinical use in cardiovascular nuclear medicine.

Radiopharmaceuticals for Nuclear Cardiology

The clinically useful cardiac imaging procedures using radionuclides fall into one of four categories:
1. The assessment of ventricular function.
2. The assessment of the coronary circulation based on coronary perfusion.
3. The diagnosis of myocardial ischemia and acute myocardial infarction (AMI).
4. Intracardiac shunt studies.

Some common clinical applications and the associated radiodiagnostic agents are shown in Table 3-3.

TABLE 3-3
Radiodiagnostic Agents and Clinical Applications

Type of Study	Imaging Technique	Classification of Agent	Radiotracers Employed
Diagnosis of acute myocardial infarction	MVSS	Infarct Avid	^{99m}Tc-pyrophosphate and diphosphonates; ^{99m}Tc-glucoheptonate°; ^{197m}Hg-hydroxymercurifluorescein
	MVSS	Normal myocardium, localizing agent extractable, diffusable indicators	^{201}Tl (thallous ion) ^{43}K, ^{82}Rb, ^{129}Cs, ^{13}NH$_3$, ^{11}C-palmitic acid°, ^{123}I-fatty acids°, ^{13}N-asparagine°
Detection and evaluation of coronary artery disease	MVSS Stress Test	Normal myocardium, localizing agents, freely diffusable non-diffusion limited	Same as above ^{133}Xe, ^{127}Xe, ^{81}Kr
Assessment of ventricular performance	First Transit	Non-particulate	^{99m}TcO$_4^-$, ^{99m}Tc-DTPA, ^{99m}Tc-glucoheptonate, ^{99m}Tc-HSA, ^{99m}Tc-RBC
	EGAS	Intravascular Tracer	
Quantitation of Intracardiac Shunt	MVSS	Particulate Perfusion	^{113m}In-transferrin, ^{111}In-transferrin
	Right-to-left shunt	Imaging Agent	^{99m}Tc-human albumin microspheres
	First Transit Left-to-right shunt	Non-particulate	^{99m}TcO$_4^-$, ^{99m}Tc-DTPA

MVSS = Multiple view static study; EGAS = Equilibrium gated acquisition study (experimental, not in widespread use).

Radiopharmaceuticals for Analysis of Ventricular Function

Studies of ventricular function using radiopharmaceuticals are performed in two ways: (1) first pass radionuclide angiocardiography and (2) equilibrium studies.

First Pass study

The primary requirement of a radiopharmaceutical for first pass radionuclide angiocardiography is that it remains in the intravascular compartment during its first passage through the right and left cardiac chambers.

The radionuclide which has replaced ^{131}I in virtually all phases of radionuclide angiocardiography is technetium-99m. Since pertechnetate (^{99m}TcO$_4^-$) is the chemical form of ^{99m}Tc after its elution from the ^{99}Mo-^{99m}Tc-generator, it is the most readily available and least expensive of the technetium-99m pharmaceuticals. While pertechnetate leaks out rapidly into the extracellular space with an intravascular half-life of approximately one hour, it does remain intravascular during its first intracardiac transit and is used extensively for first pass studies. However, ^{99m}Tc-DTPA (diethylenetriamine pentaacetic acid) or ^{99m}Tc-glucoheptonate, can also be used for first pass studies of the heart. The major disadvantage of ^{99m}Tc is its long half-life when compared to the length of the procedure. After intravenous injection the material remains in the intravascular and extracellular spaces precluding serial studies.

One way to increase the number of serial studies is to use Tc sulfur colloid, a radiopharmaceutical extracted by the reticuloendothelial system of the liver, spleen and bone marrow within several minutes after intravenous injection.[3] The disadvantage of this method is that it exposes the radiosensitive bone marrow to a high radiation dose. Technetium-99m pyrophosphate is an attractive alternative when a first pass study is followed by acute infarct scintigraphy. The two studies can be done 90 minutes apart after a single injection of radiopharmaceutical. The use of ^{99m}Tc-DTPA and ^{99m}Tc-glucoheptonate also represents an improvement since the blood clearance and excretion of these radiopharmaceuticals is more rapid than that of ^{99m}Tc-pertechnetate, reducing the whole body radiation dose and more importantly, shortening the time between sequential studies.[4]

The development of short-lived radionuclides such as tantalum-178 (T½ = 9 minutes) will increase the flexibility of this technique.[5] Tantalum-178 is eluted from a tungsten generator (^{178}W-^{178}Ta) and can be used for imaging with different instruments. Indium-113m, eluted from a tin generator (^{113}Sn-^{113m} In), can also be used in a single probe radio-cardiography. Because photon energy is high (393 keV), tissue absorption is minimal. Since its half-life is short, (T½ = 100 minutes) studies can be repeated at 3 to 4 hour intervals. Indium-113m is not suitable for studies with scintillation cameras because of its high photon energy.

Equilibrium Studies

The radiopharmaceutical for equilibrium (ECG-gated) studies must remain in the intravascular space throughout the course of the study. If continual monitoring is anticipated, the radiopharmaceutical must remain within the intravascular space for at least one or two half-lives. ^{99m}Tc-human serum albumin (HSA) and ^{99m}Tc-tagged red blood cells have been advocated for this purpose. ^{99m}Tc-HSA is less satisfactory for gated studies for two reasons: (1) the liver space is larger than the intravascular space, increasing the background activity in the liver; (2) ^{99m}Tc HSA is cleared from the blood rapidly, precluding prolonged monitoring for cardiac studies.

Technetium-99m labeled red blood cells have slow blood clearance once the initial equilibration of the tracer has been reached. The red cells can be tagged in vivo by injecting 300 to 700 micrograms of stannous ion intravenously, followed by another injection of ^{99m}Tc-pertechnetate 15 minutes later. Approximately 60 to 80 percent of the ^{99m}Tc-pertechnetate labels the red blood cells. The remainder is excreted by the kidneys. Equilibration is reached after five minutes. Since rapid renal clearance is required for optimal studies, this technique is less satisfactory for patients with poor renal clearance which results in high background activity and poor target-to-background ratios. An alternative for which kits have been developed is the in vitro labeling of the red blood cells.[6] This technique requires manipululation of cells and takes more time than in vivo labeling, but it labels red cells with 98 percent or greater efficiency.

Radiopharmaceuticals for Assessing Myocardial Integrity

Myocardial Perfusion Studies

Potassium ions are necessary for myocardial contraction and therefore radiopotassium would be a logical biologic tracer for assessing myocardial integrity. The first potassium tracer available for human use had energies that were unsatisfactory for imaging with scintillation detectors.[7] Potassium-43 has physical characteristics more compatible with the instrumentation currently used for external imaging.[8] While results with this agent have been promising, this radiotracer is still limited by a relatively long half-life (22.4 hours) precluding serial studies; by beta emission that exposes the patient to a high absorbed radiation dose; by highly energetic photons with a photopeak at 373 keV, which makes imaging with the gamma camera difficult; and by a high photopeak at 619 keV, that scatters radiation and substantially degrades the image.

Perfusion Studies with Potassium Analogues

Other potassium analogues have been introduced including cesium-129,[9] rubidium-81,[10] and thallium-201.[11] All have advantages over [43]K. Thallium-201, a metallic element with properties similar to potassium[12,13] is the most promising. It has biological and physical characteristics well suited to myocardial perfusion scintigraphy. Thallium clears the blood as rapidly as potassium or rubidium, but it clears the myocardium more slowly so that a maximum heart-to-blood ratio is reached in 10 minutes. The distributions of thallium and rubidium throughout the left venticle are similar. Thallium appears to concentrate in myocardium (3 percent of injected dose) to a greater degree than does potassium or rubidium.[14] The extraction of thallium by the myocardium is most likely due to activation of the sodium-potassium adenosine triphosphatase (ATPase) system. Thallium appears to bind at two sites on the enzyme system compared to one site for potassium. This may account for the prolonged clearance of thallium from the myocardium.[13]

In addition to biological advantages over potassium and the other potassium analogues, thallium-201 has physical characteristics more suited to imaging with scintillation camera systems.[14] Only 10 percent of disintegrations result in gamma emmisions at 135 and 167 keV. Characteristic x-rays are given off in the range of 69 to 83 keV, and these are used for external imaging. While the use of this energy peak results in some loss of spatial resolution as a result of the difficulty in using pulse height analysis to eliminate scattered radiation from the primary photopeak, this energy range does permit imaging with scintillation cameras and enables greater resolution than is possible with either [43]K, [81]Rb, or [129]Cs.

There are several factors affecting the myocardial uptake and distribution of monovalent cations. The degree to which the distribution of these monovalent cations will reflect blood flow depends on the extraction fraction remaining constant at different flow rates.[15-17] Another factor that affects the distribution of potassium analogues is the integrity of cell membrane adenosine triphosphatase (ATPase) which maintains transmembrane electrochemical gradients of sodium and potassium.[18-20]

Perfusion During Stress in Patients with Coronary Artery Disease

When myocardial perfusion scintigraphy is done after stress, transiently ischemic myocardium can be detected.[21] Thus, regions that are perfused normally at rest but show decreased perfusion after exercise represent ischemic zones, while perfusion defects both at rest and after exercise represent zones of previous infarction. A potassium analogue (^{201}Tl) with a high extraction efficiency is injected at the time of maximal stress during either treadmill or bicycle exercise. The patient is subsequently imaged immediately after exercise and several hours of rest. The redistribution of tracer reflects the ischemia at the time of injection. Thallium-201 is well-suited for this type of study as it is cleared from the blood within one minute after injection. Since it begins to redistribute within 10 minutes after injection,[22] imaging must be done soon after injection. Thus the imaging equipment and the treadmill or bicycle should be located at the same site, and imaging should be done with a high resolution, low energy collimator. The abnormal perfusion scintigrams obtained during stress in patients with coronary artery disease are the result of a heterogeneous increase in myocardial blood flow. In normal individuals, blood flow increases uniformly during exercise or other forms of stress simulating interventions. In patients with coronary artery disease, the increase in blood flow during stress is not nearly as great, and in fact, there is an inverse relationship between the increase in flow and percent of coronary artery stenosis once the lumen is narrow as much as 40 to 50 percent.[22]

When positron-emitting potassium analogues and positron imaging devices are used in perfusion scintigraphy, the heart can be displayed in three dimensions. Because of the short half-life of these positron-emitting nuclides, a number of studies may be done under various stress states and sequential examinations performed to follow the course of ischemia or infarction. One of the more promising agents is rubidium-82, with a 75 second half-life.[23]

A number of positron-emitting radiopharmaceuticals have been used to evaluate coronary artery disease. Ammonia (^{13}NH$_3$) has been used as a marker of myocardial perfusion, and there has been a close correlation between changes in size of the resultant perfusion defect and the clinical course of patients with acute infarction.[24]

Radiopharmaceuticals for Assessing Myocardial Metabolism

Short-lived, positron-emitting radionuclides, such as oxygen-15, nitrogen-13 and carbon-11 offer advantages in the study of metabolic processes. These elements are ubiquitous in naturally occurring metabolic processes. These nuclides are the only isotopes of these elements suitable for imaging. Thus, ^{15}O and ^{13}N can be incorporated into radiopharmaceuticals that are true metabolic substrates and consequently can be tailored to the investigation of selected metabolic pathways. Since myocardial ischemia alters the myocardial metabolism of free fatty acids by decreasing oxidation and increasing conversion to triglycerides, free fatty acids labeled with positron-emitting nuclides, such as ^{11}C palmitate, may be particularly suitable for quantitative studies of myocardial metabolism.[24]

Infarct-Avid Radiopharmaceuticals

Technetium-99m Pyrophosphate

Technetium-99m (^{99m}Tc) pyrophosphate is the radiotracer of choice for imaging acute myocardial infarction in man.[25-27] Fifty percent of the injected dose is extracted by bone, and the remainder is rapidly excreted through the kidneys. At 90 minutes, less than 5 percent of the injected dose remains in the blood. The myocardial uptake of ^{99m}Tc pyrophosphate is dependent on three factors: (1) regional blood flow, (2) calcification, and (3) tissue damage.

The uptake of ^{99m}Tc pyrophosphate is directly related to the degree of tissue damage, but because the pharmaceutical must reach the damaged tissue for extraction, uptake is inversely related to the degree of flow. Following acute coronary occlusion, increased concentrations of ^{99m}Tc pyrophosphate are found in regions with only minimal reductions in blood flow.[28] The highest concentration ratios between damaged and normal myocardium occur when local blood flow is 20 percent to 40 percent of normal. As flow is reduced further the concentration ratios begin to fall until, in region of minimal flow (0 percent to 5 percent of normal), ^{99m}Tc pyrophosphate concentration may be negligible.

Buja et al.[29] found the highest ^{99m}Tc pyrophosphate concentration ratios in the outer periphery of the infarct. In 17 dogs undergoing left anterior descending artery ligation and injected 18 to 48 hours later with ^{99m}Tc pyrophosphate, the concentration of the pyrophosphate in the outer periphery zone of the infarction was 24.5 times that of normal myocardium, while the concentration in the inner periphery was 7.8 times normal. The concentration in the center of the infarct was only 1.7 times normal. Thus, the status of regional myocardial perfusion after occlusion appears to be a key determinant for the scintigraphic detection of such infarcts with pyrophosphate.

There was also a coincident correlation between the presence of contraction bands and calcium deposits and uptake of labeled pyrophosphate. Thus, numerous irreversibly injured muscle cells with contraction bands and calcium deposits were found in the outer periphery of the infarct where the pyrophosphate uptake was high; the reverse was true in the central zones of the infarct. This led the investigators to hypothesize that pyrophosphate uptake was also dependent on the presence of calcium. There is a close correlation between the subcellular distribution of ^{99m}Tc pyrophosphate and that of calcium.[30] Concentration ratios for ^{99m}Tc pyrophosphate and calcium of 11.0 ± 0.4 and 3.1 ± 0.9 were found in the border zones of the acute myocardial infarct with focal necrosis, 17.4 ± 1.9 and 16.7 ± 6.4 in peripheral zones with extensive necrosis, and 6.5 ± 1.5 and 6.2 ± 1.0 in central zones with confluent necrosis as compared to normal myocardium. There was a correlation between the uptake of pyrophosphate and calcium within subcellular fractions. These studies suggest that elevated intracellular calcium levels play a key role in myocardial scintigraphy by establishing a chemical milieu which induces extraction and concentration of ^{99m}Tc pyrophosphate. Observing that the hydroxyapatite crystals were formed within mitochondria in the peripheral zones of the acute infarct, Bonte et al. hypothesized that ^{99m}Tc pyrophosphate, a calcium chelate, is sequestered by these crystals during the acute phase of myocardial infarction.[27] Mitochondrial calcification has been detected as early as two to four hours after permanent occlusion and is clearly visible by 12 to 24 hours.[31] The calcification occurred primarily in irreversibly damaged tissue.

Recent experimental evidence suggests that, while the localization of radionuclide in the damaged myocardium may be related to the presence of calcium, the site of sequestration of the radiopharmaceutical is not the mitochondria. In studies carried out in a tissue culture model, Dewanjee found uptake of the radionuclide primarily in the soluble and nuclear fractions.[32] Only a small percentage (8.5 percent in the liver and 12.3 percent in the dead cells) was observed in the mitochondria. Other investigators have also found the highest levels in the supernate and in membrane and cell debris with the lowest concentrations in microsomes and mitochondria.[30] While pure fractionation of subcellular organelles is extremely difficult, particularly with myocardial tissue, this evidence strongly suggests that the method of localization is not mitochondrial sequestration. Other studies have also cast further doubt on the precise role of calcification in ^{99m}Tc pyrophosphate sequestration. Using a fetal mouse heart tissue culture model, Schelbert et al. showed a poor correlation between calcium and ^{99m}Tc pyrophosphate uptake during oxygen and glucose metabolism.[33] Concentration of ^{99m}Tc pyrophosphate is not proportional to the extent of infarction. In a canine model of acute infarction, there was a negative correlation between maximum radioactivity recorded in the precordial image and the extent of infarction $(r= -0.86)$.[34]

Other investigators have also found that, while pyrophosphate uptake appeared limited to histologically necrotic tissue, pyrophosphate ratios between normally perfused tissue adjacent to the ischemic segment and distant normal tissue were elevated (6.72 ± 0.4).[28,35] These investigators also found no linear relationship between the extent of necrosis and accumulation of pyrophosphate. Since the intensity of accumulation of the pyrophosphate on the infarcted scintigrams will be related to the degree of perfusion as well as the extent of necrosis, these investigators concluded that the intensity of radionuclide uptake on the myocardial scintigram cannot be used as a quantitative index of infarct size.

Technetium-99m Tetracycline

Technetium-99m (^{99m}Tc) tetracycline was the first radiopharmaceutical to demonstrate infarct avidity in man. [36,37] Initial results demonstrated that acute myocardial infarction could be detected accurately 24 hours after the radionuclide was injected.[37] This turned out to be the major limitation to its use in acute infarct scintigraphy. In addition, concentration of the tracer within the infarct is only moderately elevated and high concentration within the liver may obscure the visualization of uptake in the diaphragmatic segment of the heart. In infarcts involving less than 15 percent of the myocardium, the increase in concentration of ^{99m}Tc tetracycline is less than two times that in normal tissue.

Technetium-99m Glucoheptonate

Other radiotracers have also been used for acute infarct scintigraphy. Accumulation of ^{99m}Tc glucoheptonate within the infarcted focus has been tested in a number of animal models.[38] Following acute myocardial infarction in dogs, ratios between concentrations in infarcted and normal myocardium have ranged from 11:1 to 20:1. Uptake of radionuclide in the infarcted area occurs rapidly after coronary artery occlusion. Concentrations of approximately 21:1 can be reached in the canine model hours after infarction (four hours after the tracer is injected). The accuracy for detecting acute infarction in man with this radiotracer appears to be related to the age and size of the infarct. Rossman et al. found that 80 percent of infarcts were detected by this technique. The detection rate was highest for transmural infarcts, and lowest for subendocardial myocardial infarcts.[39] In patients with infarcts from 2 to 6 days old, only three of 13 infarcts were detected by scintigraphy.[25] Thus, while this radiotracer may be useful during the early stage of acute infarction, it is not as sensitive as ^{99m}Tc pyrophosphate after the first day.

Experimental Radiopharmaceuticals in Nuclear Cardiology

Hydroxymercurifluoresceins

Using the heat-damaged rat heart model described by Adler and his associates,[40] it has been possible to demonstrate that a large number of radiopharmaceuticals have the property of being sequestered by acutely damaged myocardium.[41] Studies with a mercury-containing compound, diiodohydroxymercurifluorescein, yield higher concentration ratios between damaged and normal myocardium than any other radiopharmaceutical tested. In addition, the percent of injected dose per gram is almost six times that of the bone-seeking radiotracers. The presence of mercury in the radiocompound has correlated strongly with its concentration in the infarct.[41] The evidence indicates strongly that both the polycyclic aromatic moiety and the hydroxymercuric group are necessary for the high selectivity that is required for imaging.

Myosin Antibody

Purified radiolabeled antibody against cardiac myosin has also been demonstrated in regions of acute infarction. After the intravenous injection of radioiodine-labeled (Fab') fragments of antibodies specific for cardiac myosin, ratios of 6.1 ± 0.6 and 3.3 ± 0.4 between infarcted and normal myocardium have been obtained in the epicardium and endocardium, respectively. There is an inverse relationship between regional myocardial blood flow and uptake of the tracer.[42] Well-defined areas of increased myocardial activity were detected 72 hours after coronary occlusion in dogs. Unfortunately, the concentration of tracer within the infarct was too low to permit imaging of the infarct within the first 24 hours after coronary occlusion. Visualization of the infarct was delayed because of the slow ciearance of tracer from the blood and poor uptake by the infarcted tissue.

Iodine-123 (^{123}I) Labeled 16-Iodo-9-Hexadecanoic Acid (IHA)

Long-chain fatty acids, an important energy source for the heart, are efficiently extracted from the blood by the myocardium. The feasibility of myocardial imaging with radioiodinated fatty acids was first demonstrated by Evans et al.[43] Labeling oleic acid with ^{131}I by saturating the double bond yields a compound of low specific activity. This compound is not extracted as efficiently as the natural unsaturated fatty acid.[44] With the recent availability of ^{123}I and the development of a radiolabeling technique to place the iodine atom on the terminal methyl group, there has been renewed interest in myocardial imaging with iodinated fatty acids.[45] The high count rates attainable with the iodine-123 label allows qualitative multiprojection images. Preliminary results from clinical studies suggest that IHA may become useful as a single agent for estimating regional myocardial perfusion and for distinguishing viable ischemic tissue from infarcted tissue.

Iodine-123 (^{123}I) Labeled β-Adrenergic Antagonists

Recent interest in using beta adrenergic antagonists to treat patients with angina and hypertension stimulated the synthesis of a great number of adrenoceptor blocking agents. One of the more commonly used agents, propranolol (Inderal) exhibits vascular or bronchial (B_2) adrenoceptor as well as cardioselective (B_1) affinity and would not be expected to give satisfactory target-to nontarget ratios between the myocardium and surrounding tissue, respectively. The more cardioselective drugs such as acebutolol and practolol have recently been radioiodinated and show promise as myocardial imaging agents.[46]

Liposomes Labeled with ^{99m}Tc DTPA

In a novel investigation, Caride and Zaret found that both positively charged and neutral liposomes containing ^{99m}Tc DTPA concentrated in infarcted regions of myocardial tissue against a flow gradient, while negative liposomes were passively distributed according to regional blood flow.[47] Liposomes can incorporate drugs in their aqueous or lipid phases and have potential as therapeutic agents. Positive and neutral liposomes may serve as vehicles for the delivery of radiodiagnostic agents to zones of infarcted myocardium having diminished blood flow.

Indium-111 (^{111}In) Labeled Leukocytes

The early inflammatory response associated with acute myocardial infarction is characterized by infiltration within 24 hours of polymorphonuclear leukocytes into regions of ischemia; this process reaches a maximum 4 to 5 days after infarction.[48] Weiss and co-workers[49] succeeded in detecting this leukocytic infiltration noninvasively in dogs. They administered autologously labeled ^{111}In leukocytes intravenously to study dogs with experimentally induced coronary occlusions. The labeled white cells accumulated in infarcted regions of the myocardium and reached maximum concentration three days after coronary occlusion. The scintigraphic studies done with the ^{111}In leukocytes correlated well with scintigram studies done with ^{13}NH$_3$. The in vivo scintigraphic studies were also verified by in vitro analysis of radioactivity in normal and infarcted myocardium.

Technetium-99m (^{99m}Tc) Labeled Heparin

Kulkarni et al. have labeled heparin with technetium-99m and documented its localization in damaged canine myocardium and coronary vessels by using models of temporary myocardial ischemia with reperfusion and fixed coronary artery occlusion.[50] Detection of damaged myocardium was possible in both modes, but the greatest concentration of ^{99m}Tc heparin in infarcted myocardium and the highest ratio of damaged-to-normal myocardial tissue were found in the reperfusion model. The data suggested that ^{99m}Tc heparin may be of value in imaging ischemic or damaged myocardium as long as significant blood flow to the damaged tissue is available.

In summary, the extent to which radiopharmaceuticals increase our ability to probe the different aspects of cardiac physiology and pathology seems enormous. At the present time, advances in radiochemistry have put radiotracers within reach of a practicing physician at a community hospital, making the noninvasive nuclear cardiology procedures available for all patients suffering from cardiac disorders.

References

1. Blumgart, H.L., and Weiss, S.: Studies on the velocity of blood flow. VII. The pulmonary circulation time in normal resting individuals. *J Clin Invest* **4**:399-425, 1927.

2. Wagner, H.N., Jr., and Emmons, H.: Characteristics of an ideal radio-pharmaceutical. In Andrews, G.A., Kniseley, R.M.,and Wagner, H.N., Jr. (Eds.): *Radioactive Pharmaceuticals*, AEC Symposium Series 6. Division of Technical Information USAFEC Conf-651111, 1966, p.5.

3. Marshall, R.C., Berger, H.J., Costin, J.C., et al.: Assessment of cardiac performance with quantitative radionuclide angiocardiography. *Circulation* **56**:820-829, 1977.

4. Ashburn, W.L., Schelbert, H.R., and Verba, J.W.: Left ventricular ejection fraction—a review of several radionuclide angiographic approaches using the scintillation camera. *Prog Cardiovasc Dis* **20**:267-284, 1978.

5. Holman, B.L., Harris, G.I., Neirinckx, R.D., et al.: Tantalum-178—a short-lived nuclide for nuclear medicine: production of the parent W-178. *J Nucl Med* **19**:510-513, 1978.

6. Richards, P.: Personal communication.

7. Bennett, K.R., Smith, R.O., Lehan, P.H., et al.: Correlation of myocardial [42]K uptake with coronary arteriography. *Radiology* **102**:117-124, 1972.

8. Hurley, P.J., Cooper, M., Reba, R.C., et al.: [43]KCl: A new radiopharmaceutical for imaging the heart. *J Nucl Med* **12**:516-519, 1971.

9. Romhilt, D.W., Adolph, R.J., Sodd, V.C., et al.: Cesium-129 myocardial scintigraphy to detect myocardial infarction. *Circulation* **48**:1242-1251, 1973.

10. Martin, N.D., Zaret, B.L., McGowan, R.L., et al.: Rubidium-81: A new myocardial scanning agent. *Radiology* **111**:651-656, 1974.

11. Lebowitz, E., Greene, M.W., Bradley-Moore, P., et al.: [201]Tl for medical use. *J Nucl Med* **14**:421-422, 1973.

12. Gehring, P.J., and Hammond, P.B.: The interrelationship between thallium and potassium in animals. *J Pharmacol Exp Ther* **55**:187-201, 1967.

13. Britten, J.S., and Blank, M.: Thallium activation of the (Na^+-K^+) - activated ATPase of rabbit kidney. *Biochem Biophys Acta* **159**:160-166, 1968.

14. Strauss, H.W., Harrison, K., Langan, J.K., et al.: Thallium-201 for myocardial imaging. Relation of thallium-201 to regional myocardial perfusion. *Circulation* **51**:641-645, 1975.

15. Becker, L., Ferreira, R., and Thomas, M.: Comparison of ^{86}Rb and microsphere estimates of left ventricular bloodflow distribution. *J Nucl Med* **15**:969-973, 1974.

16. Moir, T.W.: Measurement of coronary blood flow in dogs with normal and abnormal myocardial oxygenation and function. Comparison of flow measured by a rotameter and by Rb[86] clearance. *Circ Res* **19**:695-699, 1966.

17. Love, W.D., and Burch, G.E.: Influence of the rate of coronary plasma flow on the extraction of Rb-86 from coronary blood. *Circ Res* **7**:24-30, 1959.

18. Case, R.B.: Ion alterations during myocardial ischemia. *Cardiology* **56**:245-262, 1971.

19. Parker, J.O., Chiong, M.A., West, R.O., et al.: The effect of ischemia and alterations of heart rate on myocardial potassium balance in man. *Circulation* **42**:205-217, 1970.

20. Levenson, N.I., Adolph, R.J., Romhilt, D.W., et al.: Effect of myocardial hypoxia and ischemia on myocardial scintigraphy. *Am J Cardiol* **35**:251-257, 1975.

21. Zaret, B.L., Strauss, H. W., Martin, N.D., et al.: Noninvasive regional myocardial perfusion with radioactive potassium. Study of patients at rest, with exercise, and during angina pectoris. *N Engl J Med* **288**:809-812, 1973.

22. Schwartz, J.S., Ponto, R., Carlyle, P., et al.: Early redistribution of thallium-201 after temporary ischemia. *Circulation* **57**:332-335, 1978.

23. Budinger, T.F., Yano, Y., and Hoop, B.: A comparison of $^{82}Rb^+$ and $^{13}NH_3$ for myocardial positron scintigraphy. *J Nucl Med* **16**:429-431, 1975.

24. Weiss, E.S., Siegel, B.A., Sobel, B.E., et al.: Evaluation of myocardial metabolism and perfusion with positron-emitting radionuclides. *Prog Cardiovasc Dis* **20**:191-206, 1977.

25. Holman, B.L., Tanaka, T.T., and Lesch, M.: Evaluation of radiopharmaceuticals for the detection of acute myocardial infarction in man. *Radiology* **121**:427-430, 1976.

26. Parkey, R.W., Bonte, F.J., Meyer, S.L., et al.: A new method for radionuclide imaging of acute myocardial infarction in humans. *Circulation* **50**:540-546, 1974.

27. Bonte, F.J., Parkey, R.W., Graham, K.D., et al.: A new method for radionuclide imaging of myocardial infarcts. *Radiology* **110**:473-474, 1974.

28. Zaret, B.L., DiCola, V.C., Donabedian, R.K., et al.: Dual radionuclide study of myocardial infarction. Relationships between myocardial uptake of potassium-43, technetium-99m stannous pyrophosphate, regional myocardial blood flow and creatine phosphokinase depletion. *Circulation* **53**: 422-427, 1976.

29. Buja, L.M., Parkey, R.W., Stokely, E.M., et al.: Pathophysiology of technetium-99m stannous pyrophosphate and thallium-201 scintigraphy of acute anterior myocardial infarcts in dogs. *J Clin Invest* **57**: 1508-1522, 1976.

30. Buja, L.M., Tofe, A.J., Mukherjee, A., et al.: Role of elevated tissue calcium in myocardial infarct scintigraphy with technetium phosphorus radiopharmaceuticals. *Circulation* **54** (Suppl II): 219, 1976.

31. Shen, A.C., and Jennings, R.B.: Myocardial calcium and magnesium in acute ischemic injury. *Am J Pathol* **67**: 417-440, 1972

32. Dewanjee, M.K.: Localization of skeletal-imaging ^{99m}Tc chelates in dead cells in tissue culture: Concise communication. *J Nucl Med* **17**:993-997, 1976.

33. Schelbert, H., Ingwall, J., Sybers, H., et al.: Uptake of Tc-99m pyrophosphate (PYP) and calcium (Ca) in irreversibly damaged myocardium.

J Nucl Med **17**:534, 1976.

34. Bruno, F.P., Cobb, F.R., Rivas, F., et al.: Evaluation of [99m]Technetium stannous pyrophosphate as an imaging agent in acute myocardial infarction. *Circulation* **54**:71-78, 1976.

35. Marcus, M.L., Tomanek, R.J., Ehrhardt, J.C., et al.: Relationships between myocardial perfusion, myocardial necrosis, and technetium-99m pyrophosphate uptake in dogs subjected to sudden coronary occlusion. *Circulation* **54**:647-653, 1976.

36. Holman, B.L., Dewanjee, M.K., Idoine, J., et al.: Detection and localization of experimental myocardial infarction with ^{99m}Tc-tetracycline. *J Nucl Med* **14**:595-599, 1973.

37. Holman, B.L., Lesch, M., Zweiman, F.G., et al.: Detection and sizing of acute myocardial infarcts with [99m]Tc(Sn)tetracycline. *N Engl J Med* **291**: 159-163, 1974.

38. Rossman, D.J., Strauss, H.W., Siegel, M.E., et al.: Accumulation of ^{99m}Tc-glucoheptonate in acutely infarcted myocardium. *J Nucl Med* **16**:875-878, 1975.

39. Rossman, D.J., Rouleau, J., Strauss, H.W., et al.: Detection and size estimation of acute myocardial infarction using ^{99m}Tc-glucoheptonate. *J Nucl Med* **16**:980-985, 1975.

40. Adler, N., Camin, L.L., and Shulkin, P.: Rat model for acute myocardial infarction: Application to technetium-labeled glucoheptonate, tetracycline and polyphosphate. *J Nucl Med* **17**:203-207, 1976.

41. Davis, M.A., Holman, B.L., and Carmel, A.N.: Evaluation of radiopharmaceutical sequestered by acutely damaged myocardium. *J Nucl Med* **17**: 911-917, 1976.

42. Khaw, B.A., Beller, G.A., and Haber, E.: Experimental myocardial infarct imaging following intravenous administration of iodine-131 labeled antibody (Fab')$_2$ fragments specific for cardiac myosin. *Circulation* **57**:743-750, 1978.

43. Evans, J.R., Gunton, R.W., Baker, R.G., et al.: Use of radioiodinated fatty acid for photoscans of the heart. *Circ Res* **16**:1-10, 1964.

44. Poe, N.D., Robinson, G.D., Jr., and MacDonald, N.S.: Myocardial extraction of labeled long-chain fatty acid analogs. *Proc Soc Exper Biol Med* **148**: 215, 1975.

45. Poe, N.D., Robinson, G.D., Jr., Graham, L.S., et al.: Experimental basis for myocardial imaging with ^{123}I-labeled hexadecenoic acid. *J Nucl Med* **17**: 1077-1082, 1976.

46. Hanson, R.N., Holman, B.L., and Davis, M.A.: Synthesis and biologic distribution of radioiodinated β-adrenergic antagonists. *J Med Chem* **21**: 830, 1978.

47. Caride, V.J., and Zaret, B.L.: Liposome accumulation in regions of myocardial infarction. *Science* **198**:735-737, 1977.

48. Mallory, G.K., and White, P.D.: The speed of healing of myocardial infarction. *Am Heart J* **18**:647-671, 1939.

49. Weiss, E.S., Ahmad, S.A., Thakur, M.L., et al.: Imaging of the inflammatory response in ischemic canine myocardium with indium-111 labeled leukocytes. *Am J Cardiol* **40**:195, 1977.

50. Kulkarni, P.V., Parkey, R.W., Buja, L.M., et al.: Technetium-99m heparin: A new radiopharmaceutical to identify damaged coronary endothelium and damaged myocardium. *J Nucl Med* **19**:718,1978.

CHAPTER IV

Instrumentation for Cardiovascular Nuclear Medicine

James E. Carey, M.S., and James H. Thrall, M.D.

The special "tools" of the nuclear cardiologist are the radiopharmaceutical and the radiation detector. Cardiovascular radiopharmaceuticals are discussed in Chapter 3. The radiation detecting systems needed for cardiovascular applications of radionuclides are discussed in this chapter.

After a cardiovascular radiopharmaceutical has been administered to the patient, it localizes in the heart or cardiac blood pool in a characteristic and predictable fashion. Photons, x-rays, and/or gamma-rays are emitted as the radioactive "tag" decays. The number of photons emitted from any part of the heart or blood pool is proportional to the amount of radioactivity localized in that region. The function of the radiation detecting system is to translate the photon flux emanating from the heart into clinically useful information. For example, after ^{99m}Tc-labeled red-blood cells are administered, the photon flux per unit time is measured and the data are used to generate left ventricular time/activity curves from which information on changing heart chamber volume is inferred. The spatial distribution of the emitted photons is mapped after thallium-201 has been administered. These "maps" or images provide information on myocardial perfusion and viability. The complexity of the radiation detecting system required depends upon the type of information to be extracted from the photon flux.

The Heart as a Source of Photons

The flux of photons arriving at a radiation detector is assumed to be proportional to the number of photons emitted in the heart. This assumption would be strictly valid only if the heart were a point radiation source in air. However, this is not the case and there are several factors that distort the photon flux presented to the radiation detector. For example, "good" photons are removed from the flux (attenuation), thereby reducing information content; and "bad" photons are added to the flux (activity from surrounding tissue), thereby adding noise to the image and degrading its quality.

In all nuclear imaging procedures many potentially useful photons are removed before they reach the detector by attenuation in body tissue. The attenuation (Fig. 4-1A) involves two types of interaction: (1) absorption, where the photon transfers all of its energy to tissue and disappears before reaching the detector, and (2) scatter, where the photon transfers part of its energy to tissue, then the lower energy photon travels at an angle away from the detector. Attenuation is difficult to correct but is constant for a given patient/detector geometry and photon energy. In practice, attenuation has not been shown to significantly distort patient data and its main effect is the stealing of useful photons.

As noted above, unwanted photons are added to the flux in two ways. In all cardiological studies, the tissues in front of, behind, and beside the heart also contain radioactivity that will emit photons which travel directly to the detector (Figure 4-1B). These "bad" photons contribute to "background noise" that can distort the data from the patient and must be corrected in quantitative analysis or, in some cases, eliminated to aid interpretation of images. Various approaches for selecting restrictive regions of interest within the detector field of view and selecting background region for data correction will be discussed below with respect to the specific radiation detecting system.

"Bad" photons also arise from another source. Just as potentially useful photons can scatter out of the detector field of view, photons originating in tissue outside the detector field of view can interact with body tissue and be scattered internally at an angle that allows them to reach the detector (Fig. 4-1C). Scatter photons also cause distortion and must be removed if possible before contributing to the recorded image data. Fortunately, such photons can be distinguished from "good" photons on the basis of the photon's energy level. All of the radiation detection devices to be discussed below include electronic components designed to eliminate these unwanted scattered photons.

Radiation Detection Systems

Overview

Radiation detecting systems used in nuclear cardiology employ com-

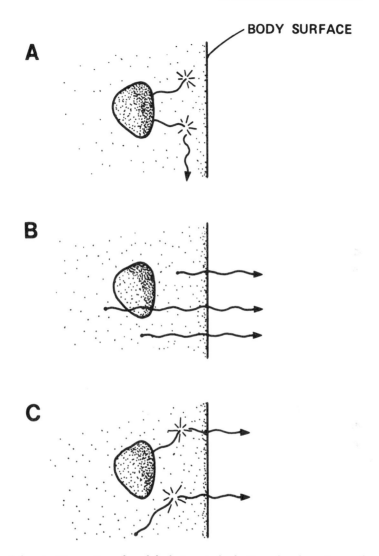

Figure 4-1. *A*, Attenuation of useful photons in body tissue by absorption and scatter. *B*, Unwanted photons from activity present in surrounding tissue. *C*, Unwanted photons scattered into the detector's field of view.

ponents that perform three basic functions: (1) a collimator which geometrically defines the tissue volume from which photons can be accepted, (2) a detector which interacts with the incoming photons and transforms absorbed photon energy into voltage pulses and (3) a recording system capable of displaying the data numerically or as an image for clinical interpretation. In all commercially available radiation detecting systems suitable for cardiological applications the collimators are made

of lead and the detectors are composed of crystalline sodium iodide
optically coupled to one or more photomultiplier tubes. All detector
systems come with a wide variety of display and recording options.

Collimators

A bare sodium iodide crystal will accept photons from all directions
(Fig. 4-2A). The function of the lead collimator is to limit the field of
view of the sodium iodide crystal to a specific tissue volume in the
patient. To do so, the collimator absorbs photons approaching the crystal

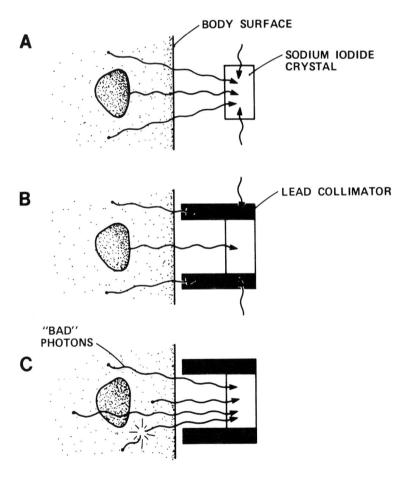

Figure 4-2. *A*, Unshielded sodium iodide crystal accepts photons from all directions. *B*,
Collimated sodium iodide crystal limits field of view to a specific tissue volume reducing
background contribution. *C*, Even with collimation, background photons can still reach
detector.

at the wrong angles (Fig. 4-2*B*). Lead is the most commonly used collimator material because of its excellent properties of photon absorption at the photon energies used, relatively low cost, and ease of fabrication. Unfortunately, the field of view defined by the collimator allows some "bad" photons to reach the detector (Fig. 4-2*C*) and, as mentioned above, other means are used to eliminate these photons.

Detector

The radiation detecting medium most commonly employed is crystalline sodium iodide (NaI) chosen for its good properties as a scintillator. By definition a scintillator is a substance that transforms x- and gamma ray energy into visible light energy. Although pure sodium iodide is not a good scintillator at room temperature, sodium iodide that has been contaminated with thallium iodide impurities [NaI(Tl)] during crystal growth scintillates efficiently at room temperature, emitting light in the ultraviolet-blue region of the electromagnetic spectrum. Sodium iodide has a relatively high effective atomic number and absorbs photons readily for the photon energies commonly employed clinically. The light flash emitted by the crystal is detected by an electronic device called a photomultiplier tube (PMT). The PMT transforms visible light energy into an electrical pulse (Fig. 4-3). Although this multi-step process of converting photon energy into electrical energy may seem rather complicated, it is the most efficient means currently available and provides electrical signals suitable for further processing.

The presence of the electrical signal (voltage pulse) at the output of the PMT indicates that an x- or gamma ray has interacted with the sodium

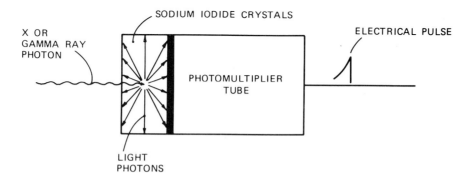

Figure 4-3. Basic crystal-PMT combination that transforms X- or gamma ray photon energy into an electrical pulse.

iodide crystal. In addition, pulse height is porportional to the photon energy absorbed in the crystal. The greater the energy absorbed, the taller the pulse (Fig. 4-4). This fact allows not only the detection of x-and gamma ray photons, but the selection of specific pulse heights of interest corresponding to the energy of unscattered photons. An electronic device called a "pulse height analyzer" is incorporated into the radiation detecting systems to achieve this end. Electrical pulses generated by the crystal/PMT combination pass into the pulse height analyzer. Pulses within the acceptable range cause the pulse height analyzer to generate "logic" pulses that are in turn used to trigger the storage and/or display devices. Thus, the pulse height analyzer is used to eliminate unwanted scattered photons from being recorded. These photons have less energy than the "good" photons and result in PMT output pulses too low to generate a logic pulse.

The Cardiac Probe

The simplest radiation detection system used in nuclear cardiology is the cardiac probe. In this system (Fig. 4-5), the collimator is basically a hollow lead cylinder consisting of one large hole surrounded by a lead

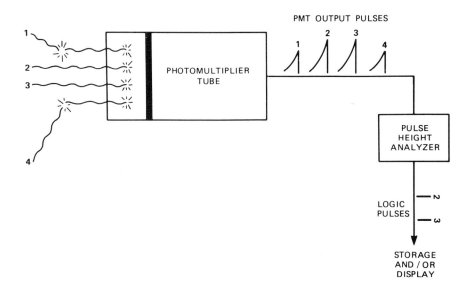

Figure 4-4. Crystal-PMT combination with pulse height analyzer to eliminate scattered photons. Photons 1 and 4 have been scattered in tissue before reaching detector. Scattered photons have less energy than "good" photons resulting in smaller PMT output pulses that are eliminated by the pulse height analyzer.

sleeve. The crystal is typically a right cylinder, 2 inches in diameter and 2 inches thick, viewed by a single photomultiplier tube. A pulse height analyzer is incorporated to eliminate scatter radiation. This cardiac probe also incorporates a fast response count rate meter that reads out onto a strip chart recorder.

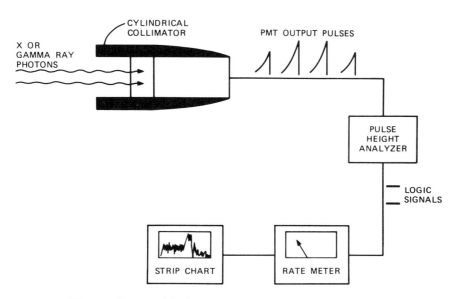

Figure 4-5.   Simplified schematic diagram of the cardiac probe.

The principal advantage of the single hole collimator design is one of sensitivity. The collimator defines a field of view that includes the heart and surrounding tissue. Photons emitted from within this field of view and traveling toward the detector "see" very little lead on their way to the detector. This allows a large photon flux to reach the detector and yields high count rate data. Photons emitted outside of the field of view and traveling at wrong angles are stopped by the collimator. Photons outside the field of view, but scattered to the detector are eliminated by the pulse height analyzer.

The major limitation of the cardiac probe is the lack of spatial resolution and, therefore, it cannot be used for heart imaging. However, the components found in the cardiac probe system are at the "heart" of all instruments used in nuclear cardiology (and in nuclear medicine in general). The collimator may be more sophisticated, the detector larger, the PMT's many, and the display and readout device more advanced, but the basic functions of definition, detection, pulse height analysis, and display are still there.

The field of view of early cardiac probe systems encompassed a major portion of the heart, resulting in extremely complex radiocardiograms from which only gross patterns could be recognized. Newly designed collimators restrict the field of view to a more specific region of interest within the heart and allow better determination of background counts for data correction. A more recent version of this approach incorporates two detectors into a single cardiac probe. A central collimated detector determines left ventricular activity while the annular detector is collimated to record background activity simultaneously from the same radiotracer injection.

The advantages and disadvantages of the cardiac probe system are summarized in Table 4-1. Advantages include relatively low cost, mobility for bedside data collection, and superior sensitivity, up to 20,000 counts per second from 1 to 1.15 millicuries of ^{99m}Tc-labeled serum albumin. Disadvantages include the inability to produce an image and/or to obtain data from smaller subregions of the heart. The primary technical difficulty associated with this probe technique is positioning the detector accurately so that the desired cardiac chamber can be identified. However, ultrasonic and radiographic means have been used to improve the accuracy of probe placement over the heart.

The Anger Camera

The most commonly used radiation detection system for nuclear cardiology is the Anger-type gamma camera. The unique feature that characterizes an "Anger camera" is the combination of a single, large, thin, right-cylindrical sodium iodide crystal viewed by a hexagonal array of photomultiplier tubes (37 to 91 tubes on recent generation systems) (Fig. 4-6). Light photons emitted when x or gamma ray energy is absorbed in the crystal are "seen" by the PMT array. The photomultiplier tubes closest to the point of absorption receive more light photons than those further away. The greater the number of light photons striking the face of a given PMT, the larger its output pulse. Thus, individual PMT output pulses are sent to an analog position computer. The position computer takes all the output pulses, analyzes their heights, and generates x, y positioning signals that represent the Cartesian coordinates of the point within the crystal where the photon was absorbed. These x, y signals are then channeled to two different electronic pathways. Following one path, the x, y signals (voltage pulses) are added together to form a so-called "Z" pulse. The height of this pulse is proportional to the output from all of the PMT's and, therefore, to the

TABLE 4-1
Advantages and Disadvantages of Radiation Detecting Systems Used for Nuclear Cardiology

Advantages	Disadvantages
CARDIAC PROBE SYSTEM	
Low cost	Non-image forming
Greatest mobility	Global LVF only
High sensitivity	Accurate Positioning difficult
ANGER-SINGLE CRYSTAL CAMERA	
Image forming	Average cost
Best image resolution	Technical skill required
Mobile systems available	Lowest count rates
MULTI-CRYSTAL CAMERA	
Image forming	High cost
Computer mandatory	No mobile capability
High sensitivity	Limited pulse height resolution
	Limited spatial resolution
	(in dynamic imaging)

total energy absorbed in the crystal. Thus, the "Z" pulse is used for pulse height analysis in eliminating pre-detector scatter. Simultaneously, the x, y pulses are sent to the x, y input of the storage and/or display device to be used in image formation provided that the pulse height analyzer decides the signals came from a "good" photon.

The type of collimator most commonly used with the Anger camera consists of a parallel array of circular, square, or triangular holes formed in a lead matrix (typically 15,000 holes for collimators used for nuclear cardiology). Specific collimators are designed for imaging low, medium, or high energy photons. Collimators designed for use with low energy photons have less lead between the holes (that is, thinner septae) than collimators designed for use with higher energy photons. If a collimator designed for low energy photons is used with higher energy photons, the collimator septae are penetrated by off-angle photons. Septal penetration degrades the imaging data. For a given photon energy, one can choose collimators designed for high spatial resolution or for high sensitivity or for a compromise between the two. The latter are often referred to as "all purpose" collimators.

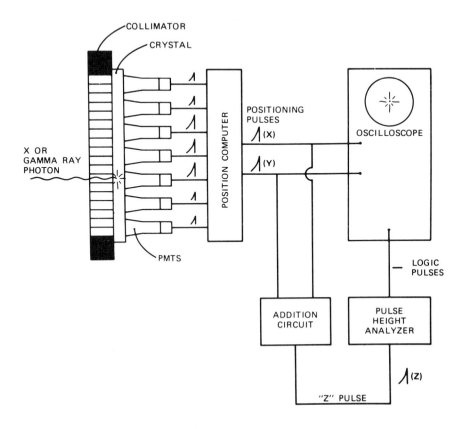

Figure 4-6. Simplified schematic diagram of the Anger-type camera.

In collimator design (Fig. 4-7A), small diameter holes result in higher spatial resolution but at the sacrifice of sensitivity. Large diameter holes (Fig. 4-7B), result in higher sensitivity but at the sacrifice of resolution. (Again, consider the probe collimator with a single, large hole and no image forming capabilities.) For a given size and number of holes, a thick collimator provides higher resolution, at depth than a thinner one (Fig. 4-7C).

For these parallel multi-hole collimators, spatial resolution decreases with increasing distance from the collimator face. Therefore, for the best spatial resolution, the collimator must be placed as close to the heart as possible. When a parallel hole collimator is angled with respect to the body surface in order to provide a view of the heart from a more advantageous angle (e.g., oblique views of the heart or caudal tilt), the average distance of the collimator from the heart is increased, resulting in a loss of spatial resolution. In order to obtain these advantageous angles, but still keep the collimator flat against the body surface, two

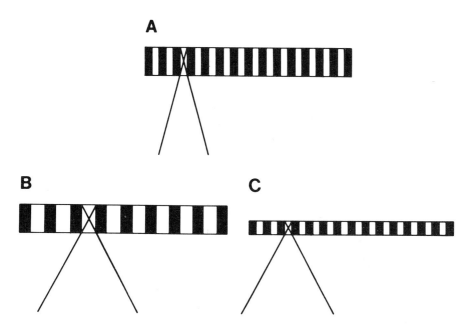

Figure 4-7. *A*, Parallel multi-hole collimator. Small diameter holes result in narrow field of view (small cone). This provides high resolution but low sensitivity. *B*, Sensitivity increased by larger diameter holes or, *C*, by thinner collimator (at the cost of spatial resolution, however).

modifications, of the parallel hole collimator have been suggested for cardiac imaging: the single, slant-hole collimator, and the double, slant-hole collimator. With the single-slant hole collimator, holes are fabricated parallel to each other, but at a 30° slant to the collimator surface. This design enables one to image the heart at a 30° angle left anterior oblique (LAO), right anterior oblique (RAO), and 30° caudal tilt while maintaining the collimator flat against the body surface and thus minimizing the average distance from the organ of interest. A +30°, –30° collimator (bifocal collimator) has also been designed so that simultaneous views can be taken 60° apart while the collimator is held flat against the body surface. Another variation of collimator design is the converging-hole collimator. This collimator takes advantage of the available crystal surface area. The angles available for photon acceptance are greater than with the parallel hole collimator. Sensitivity is increased and, in addition, the image is spread over a larger crystal surface area (magnification). This inherent magnification helps preserve spatial resolution with somewhat better depth than is possible with a parallel hole collimator. Although there is some image distortion due to unequal magnification at different depths, this collimator has been used successfully for static myocardial perfusion and infarct imaging.

Commercially available cameras have crystals that provide fields of view from 10 inches in diameter to 16 inches in diameter. The standard field of view systems have 10 inch diameters and the 15 to 16 inch diameter field of view systems are referred to as wide or large field of view systems. Even the 10 inch field of view is larger than necessary for heart imaging and the entire crystal detecting surface area is not used to full advantage with the parallel hole collimators. Crystal thickness is typically ½ inch, although some newer systems may have crystals as thin as ¼ inch. Thinner crystals result in a higher spatial resolution image due to better light photon collection at the PMT's. The thinner crystals sacrifice sensitivity due to the lower probability of x- or gamma ray photon absorption in the thinner crystal. The ¼ inch thickness is quite adequate for technetium-99m and thallium-201 which are the two most important radionuclides used in cardiologic studies, but offers low sensitivity at higher energies (e.g., iodine-131 photons).

The x, y positioning signals are usually applied to the deflection plates of an oscilloscope cathode ray tube (CRT). The deflection plates position the CRT's electron beam to a point on the display phosphor corresponding to the point of absorption of the photon in the sodium iodide crystal. Images are obtained by exposing the photographic emulsion (polaroid or transparency film) to the light flashes occurring in the phosphor.

The relative advantages and disadvantages of the Anger-type camera are summarized in Table 4-1. The main advantage of this system is its ability to obtain an image. The image quality of the Anger-type cameras has improved dramatically over the past several years and these systems provide excellent spatial resolution for both static and dynamic heart imaging and have pulse height resolution (ability to reject scatter) approaching that of the cardiac probe systems.

Dedicated minicomputer and microcomputer systems are available from a number of manufacturers for use with Anger cameras. These computers have extensive software packages for performing and analyzing cardiological studies. Mobile camera-computer systems have been introduced recently that allow a full range of studies to be performed and analyzed at the bedside.

Over the past 10 years, Anger-type cameras have become the single most widely used imaging device in nuclear medicine. They can be easily modified to perform all current clinical procedures required in nuclear cardiology. The relative disadvantages of the system are cost (approximately $110,000 to $117,000 for the camera-computer combination versus $25,000 for the most expensive cardiac probe system) and the increased technical skills necessary (on the part of both physician and technologist) for effective operation of the system. In addition, although much improved over the earlier generation cameras, the count rate sensitivity of the Anger-type camera is less than that of the cardiac probe systems and the multi-crystal camera (next section), resulting in limited counting rates, especially for first-pass studies.

Multi-Crystal Gamma Camera

The major alternative to the Anger single crystal gamma camera is the computerized multi-crystal camera. This system is characterized by a detector that contains 294 small, discrete sodium iodide crystals rather than one large crystal as does the Anger camera. Light photons emitted as x- and gamma ray photons are absorbed in the crystals and are transmitted by a relatively long Plexiglas light pipe array to the photomultiplier tubes. Each "good" photon event that occurs in a crystal results in a number recorded in computer memory. The location in memory corresponds to that of the absorbing crystal in the detector array (Fig. 4-8).

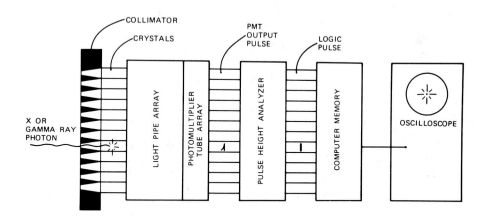

Figure 4-8. Simplified schematic diagram of the multi-crystal gamma camera.

The parallel-hole lead collimators used in the multi-crystal camera are constructed of square, tapered holes. The collimators are made of three slabs, that allow total collimator thickness of either 1.0, 1.5, or 2.5 inches corresponding to coarse-, medium-, and high-resolution collimators, respectively. Each individual crystal has a square face $5/16$ inch on a side and is 1.5 inches thick. The crystals are arranged in a 14×21 rectangular array that provides a field of view of 6×9 inches.

The advantages and disadvantages of the multi-crystal gamma camera are summarized in Table 4-1. Like the Anger-type gamma camera, the multi-crystal camera is capable of both static and dynamic imaging. The system incorporates an on-line computer for data acquisition, storage, manipulation and display. It can be used to evaluate heart function on both a global and regional basis. The multi-crystal camera has excellent count rate capabilities (up to 400,000 counts per second from recent generation systems[*]). This high count rate allows high temporal resolution and is particularly advantageous for the first pass studies.

The disadvantages of the system are cost (approximately $180,000) and the technical skill necessary for effective system operation. The multi-crystal camera is not mobile and therefore cannot be brought to the patient's bedside. The long light pipe arrangement results in a limited pulse height resolution and the spatial resolution is inferior to that of the Anger camera.

The multi-crystal camera was introduced into nuclear medicine at about the same time as the Anger-type camera (early 1960's). The Anger camera evolved into the "bread and butter" radiation detecting system of the nuclear medicine laboratory. The multi-crystal camera has not been as well accepted for general nuclear medicine work. The ability to perform "first-pass" radionuclide angiography has given new life to the multi-crystal camera because of its high count rate capabilities.

Computers

Dedicated minicomputers have become an integral part of many nuclear cardiological procedures and are a sine qua non for multiframe gated blood pool imaging. The computer is valuable for cardiological studies because of its unique capacity to acquire and store data with high spatial and temporal resolution, thereby providing a means for analyzing the data quantitatively and displaying it in enhanced and dynamic formats. During computer processing, the integrity of the raw data is preserved allowing use of multiple analytic and/or display options. From a hardware standpoint, the physical components of computers used in nuclear medicine are similar to those used in other applications (Fig. 4-9). However, all commercial vendors of computers used in nuclear medicine have developed special software programs for acquiring, analyzing and displaying cardiological studies. These programs are discussed in the following chapter.

---

[*]System Seventy-Seven, Baird Atomic, Inc.

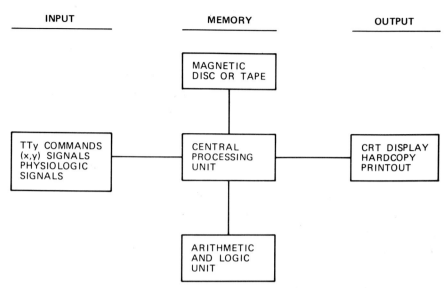

Figure 4-9. Physical components of nuclear medicine computer (hardware).

Creation of the Digital Image

The x and y analog pulses generated by Anger-type camera position circuitry are not compatible with computers, and in order to be accepted by the computer these signals must first be digitized. To accomplish this, a device called an "analog to digital converter" (ADC) is interfaced between the gamma camera and computer. The ADC's (1 for x and 1 for y position signals) produce binary numbers corresponding to the magnitude of the x, y voltage pulses. To be recorded in the computer memory, the corresponding Z pulse must indicate that the photon was a "good" photon.

Two fundamentally different modes of storing digitized data are in current use: list mode and frame (histogram) mode. In some respects list mode is simpler. Each pair of digitized x, y position signals is stored in one word of a computer's memory. The storage is sequential. Since list mode acquisition simply represents a line of data flowing into the computer memory, data other than the position coordinate pairs can be intermixed for future data formatting. For example, time markers or physiologic signals can be recorded. With the x, y pairs permanently stored in the computer memory, images can be built up in a variety of ways while preserving the original data. This flexibility is advantageous but the memory storage requirements of list mode acquisition are formidable, since each event occupies a computer word and the reformatting process generally requires several minutes before an image can be built up.

In the alternative frame mode approach, the digitized x, y pairs are used to create an image that may be thought as a matrix superimposed on the analog data (Fig. 4-10). The x and y numbers generated by the ADC's are sent to a device in the camera computer interface called an address maker. The address given to each x, y pair corresponds to a particular location in the computer memory, that is to the specific matrix element which represents the closest approximation to the location of the original event. After the data has been collected, the number recorded at each matrix location equals the number of photons occurring at the corresponding location (Fig. 4-10). These numbers are then used directly for quantitative analysis and are also used to modulate the intensity of the computer display. From the diagram in Figure 4-10 it is clear that photons interacting close to each other in the gamma camera crystal are recorded as having occurred at the same location for purposes of the digital image. Large matrices provide better resolution but require more computer memory and subsequent manipulations require more time. In current practice, dynamic studies are usually acquired in 32 × 32 or 64 × 64 matrix arrays and static images in 64 × 64 or 128 × 128 matrix arrays.

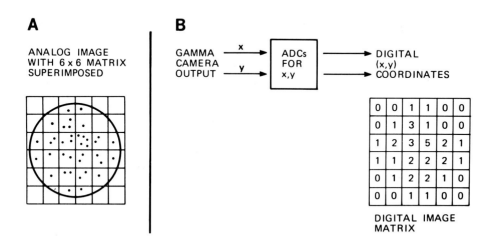

Figure 4-10. Digital Image Concept. Each photon recorded in the analog image (A) has a unique location. The number appearing at each location in the digital image (B) equals the number of photon events occurring within the boundaries of each respective matrix or picture element (pixel).

Data Analysis

The first step in quantitative cardiac image analysis is to define the geometric limits of the heart or blood pool. "Regions of interest" can be defined using a light pen and the computer scope or when the exact shape of the region is not a critical factor, rectangular regions may be defined using cursor lines. In some of the newer software programs the operator defines an expectation window and the computer automatically or semi-automatically defines regions of interest using thresholding and/or gradient techniques. The goal of the region of interest approach is to isolate the diagnostically important structures in the image and to determine the concentration of radiotracer in the defined region. For example, in the case of radionuclide ventriculography, the net radioactivity concentrated in the ventricular blood pool is proportional to ventricular volume. By defining a left ventricular region of interest at each point in the cardiac cycle and calculating the net activity emanating from it, a time activity curve can be generated which is analogous to time volume curves derived from contrast ventriculography. These curves are used for calculation of the left ventricular ejection fraction, fractional ejection rates and other quantitative parameters. In the case of thallium imaging, scans showing uptake of the tracer in certain portions of the myocardium may be compared quantitatively. Scans taken in each of these regions at different points in time, such as immediately following stress and several hours later, might also be compared. Quantitative analysis aids in diagnostic accuracy and reproducibility in addition to providing information not otherwise available.

Data Display

In analog imaging, display factors must be determined before a study begins. Frequently because of differences in patient anatomy, or drifts in response of electronic image forming circuitry, analog images are suboptimal. When data is acquired in digital form on the computer, image parameters may be optimized retrospectively in each scan. In addition, simple manipulations may nhance the images. For example, in most cardiac images the target-to-background ratio does not exceed 2:1 or 3:1 and subtraction of extra cardiac background activity may improve visualization of heart structures. More sophisticated processing called "filtering" is also being used to enhance images.

Perhaps a more important use of the computer for display purposes is in creating dynamic or cinematic displays. In radionuclide ventriculography, it is extremely useful to create a closed loop of a multi-frame sequence of images corresponding to a representative heart cycle. The endless movie loop may then be relayed at real-time rate equal to the patient's heart rate or other arbitrary rate, much as a contrast cineangiogram can be played and replayed. The dynamic display is used for analyzing regional wall motion and assessing overall ventricular performance.

Ancillary Equipment for Cardiological Studies

In addition to the detection system and computers described above, there are a number of other devices necessary for performing certain nuclear cardiological studies. In radionuclide ventriculography, performed by the equilibrium blood pool method (see Chapter 13), a "physiologic synchronizer" or cardiac "gate" is required, and there are now a number of satisfactory devices available commercially. The purpose of the physiologic synchronizer is to provide a signal that the computer can use as a starting reference point for data collection. Typically the R wave of the ECG is used. The R wave corresponds to electrical end-diastole which is a useful starting point in the cardiac cycle. The R wave is usually a relatively high voltage, clearly defined signal.

The other major ancillary device finding increasing use in nuclear cardiology is the bicycle ergometer. Ergometers are required for radionuclide ventriculography during exercise and again there are acceptable devices commercially available. Ergometers are calibrated in either watts or KPM per minute and the commercial devices developed for cardiological applications have variable work load settings. More sophisticated ergometers are equipped with heart rate sensors and feedback circuits to achieve preset heart rate by automatically varying the work load. From an imaging standpoint, the additional key requirement for the ergometer is that the patient be able to pedal while under the gamma camera without hindrance to leg motion. The ergometer must be properly calibrated and have an accurate RPM range.

Conclusion

It is clear from the above discussions that nuclear cardiology is heavily commited to highly sophisticated instrumentation. The past decade has seen advances in detector electronics resulting in reduced dead time and increased detector sensitivity and spatial resolution. The dedicated nuclear medicine minicomputer has emerged as an indispensible device. The clinician or technologist performing cardiological studies must be familiar with the instrumentation involved since its proper utilization directly affects the quality and accuracy of the studies obtained.

Future developments will undoubtedly include further improvement in instrumentation performance. New generations of computer systems are being developed and tested, and it is entirely possible that completely new devices will be developed specifically for cardiological studies. For example, a reduced field of view gamma camera with smaller crystal and ultra-fast electronics would be useful for cardiological studies and potentially more mobile than current systems.

References

1. Rollo, F.D.: Nuclear Medicine Physics, Instrumentation, and Agents. St. Louis, C.V. Mosby, 1977.
2. Hine, G.J.: Instrumentation in Nuclear Medicine, Vol. 1. New York, Academic Press, 1967.
3. Hine, G.J. and Sorenson, J.A.: Instrumentation in Nuclear Medicine, Vol. 2. New York, Academic Press, 1974.
4. Lieberman, D.E.: Computer Methods: The Fundamentals of Digital Nuclear Medicine. St. Louis, C.V. Mosby, 1977.
5. Adelstein, S.J., Jansen, C., and Wagner, H.N., Jr.: Report of the Inter-Society Commission for Heart Disease Resources. Optimal Resource Guidelines for Radioactive Tracer Studies of the Heart and Circulation. *Circulation* **52**, 1975.
6. Holman, B.L., Sonnenblick, E.J., and Lesch, M.: Principles of Cardiovascular Nuclear Medicine. New York, Grune & Stratton, 1978.
7. Steele, P.P., Van Dyke, K., Trow, R.S., et al.: A simple and safe bedside method for serial measurement of left ventricular ejection fraction, cardiac output, and pulmonary blood volume. *Br Heart J* 36:122-131, 1974.
8. Brendt, T., Alderman, E.L., Wasnich, R., et al.: Evaluation of portable radionuclide method for measurement of left ventricular ejection fraction and cardiac output. *J Nucl Med* **16**:289-292, 1975.
9. Groch, M.W., Gottlieb, S., Hallon, S.M. et al.: A new dual-probe system for rapid bedside assessment of left ventricular function. *J Nucl Med* **17**:930-936, 1976.

10. Murphy, P., Arsenau, R., Maxon, E., et al.: Clinical significance of scintillation camera electronics capable of high processing rates. *J Nucl Med* **18**:175-179, 1977.

CHAPTER V

Relationship Of Myocardial Perfusion
To Coronary Artery Anatomy

Virinderjit S. Bamrah, M.D.,
Jagmeet S. Soin, M.D.,
and Harold L. Brooks, M.D.

To understand the significance of perfusion abnormalities in the myocardium, it is important to visualize the anatomy of the coronary arteries and the myocardial segments they perfuse. Selective coronary arteriography is the best method for delineating human coronary anatomy as well as for detecting coronary atherosclerosis in the large caliber coronary arteries. However, this technique only defines the anatomic characteristics of the obstructive atherosclerotic lesions in the coronary arteries and gives little information about the blood flow distal to obstruction in the coronary arterial tree. Myocardial perfusion imaging thus complements the coronary arteriogram by furnishing important information about myocardial blood flow. Many recent studies have demonstrated close correlation between a significant obstruction in a major coronary artery and perfusion defects in the myocardium supplied by the artery.[1,2]

Coronary Artery Anatomy

James[3] and Fulton[4] have furnished excellent descriptions of the arteries to the human heart. The two major coronary arteries usually arise from their respective sinuses of Valsalva in the proximal ascending aorta. These are shown schematically in Figure 5-1 with their respective regions of perfusion.

61

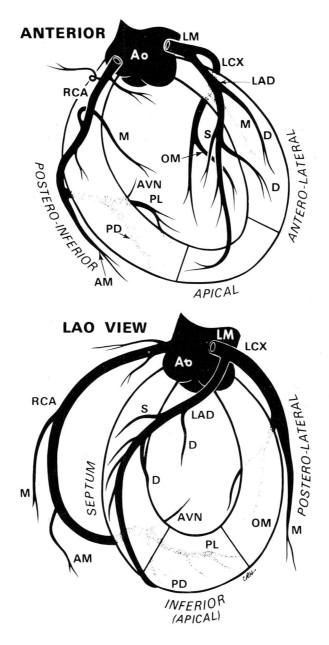

Figure 5-1.   Schematic diagram illustrating the spatial anatomy of coronary arteries and their respective regions of supply in the left ventricle as visualized in anterior and left anterior oblique views (LAO). Abbreviations: AO = aorta; RCA = right coronary artery; M = marginal; AM = acute marginal; PD = posterior descending; AVN = atrioventricular nodal; LM = left main; LAD = left anterior descending; D = diagonal; S = septal; OM = obtuse marginal; LCX = left circumflex.

Right Coronary Artery (RCA)

After arising from the aorta the RCA courses in the atrioventricular groove, bends around the acute margin of the right ventricle and continues up to or past the crux of the heart proximally. It gives a rise to a conus branch which supplies the right ventricular outflow tract. In 55 percent of individuals, the RCA gives off a sinus node artery. A variable number of marginal or right ventricular branches arise from RCA. Both the conus and acute marginal branches may make important anastamoses with the left anterior descending branches. In the majority of subjects (85 percent), RCA also supplies the atrioventricular nodal artery at the crux and then turns sharply downward toward the apex traveling in the posterior interventricular groove as a posterior descending artery (PDA). The RCA thus supplies the posterior third of the interventricular septum. Beyond the crux and origin of PDA, RCA gives off one to three posterolateral branches which supply the inferoposterior portion of the left ventricular free wall.

Left Main Coronary Artery (LMCA)

After arising from the aorta the LMCA travels downward a short distance (1 to 2 cm) before bifurcating into the left anterior descending and left circumflex arteries. Occasionally a third vessel (intermediate branch) arises from the LMCA and it perfuses the anterolateral surface of the left ventricle.

Left Anterior Descending Artery (LAD)

After arising from the LMCA, it curves gently downward into the anterior interventricular groove to the apex. In most subjects it extends just to the apex anastomosing with branches of the PDA. It gives three to six septal perforator branches which perfuse the anterior two-thirds of the interventricular septum, forming an important potential anastomotic network with perforating septal branches from the PDA. Several diagonal branches arise from the LAD and supply the anterolateral free wall of the left ventricle.

Left Circumflex Artery (LCX)

This artery arises at an angle from the LMCA and follows the left atrioventricular groove terminating a variable distance from the crux. An average of three marginal branches arise perpendicularly from the LCX and are distributed downward over the lateral and posterolateral free wall of the left ventricle. The largest of these branches is usually referred to as the obtuse marginal branch. Distally the LCX may divide into two or three posterolateral branches. In about 10 percent of the subjects, it is the dominant coronary artery and as such extends all the way to the crux, giving rise to the PDA and atrioventricular nodal branch. LCX supplies the sinus node artery in approximately 45 percent of subjects.

Anastomotic channels ranging from 100 to several hundred micrometers (μm) in diameter have been demonstrated in the normal human heart. They are most abundant in the interventricular septum, between sinus nodal and other atrial branches, between the epicardial surfaces of the right and left ventricles, cardiac apex and crux of the heart. The collaterals on the epicardial surface are much larger than those of the subendocardial regions. Under normal conditions these channels are nonfunctional and are not visualized on angiography. How they begin to support viable myocardium is not clearly understood although it appears that myocardial hypoxia, induced by significant coronary arterial stenoses, and interarterial pressure gradients are important stimulating factors.

Segmental Anatomy and Myocardial Perfusion

The left ventricular wall may be arbitrarily divided into several segments based on distribution of coronary arteries detailed above. These segments as seen by radionuclide perfusion images are illustrated schematically in Figure 5-1. While many views have been tested experimentally, the current state of the art indicates that the anterior, left anterior oblique at 45° and 60° yield the best information for evaluating a myocardial perfusion image (Figures 5-1 and 5-2). The 45° left anterior oblique (LAO) view provides maximal separation between the right and left ventricles and demonstrates best the septal, posterolateral, and inferior left ventricular segments in horizontal hearts. In patients whose hearts are vertical, the apical segment is visualized instead of inferior segment at 45° LAO view. Horizontal or vertical orientation of the heart in the chest can be easily determined by examining the anterior view. Then the segments in 45° LAO view can be appropriately named.

The LAD artery perfuses the anterolateral, septal and apical segments. The LAD lesions proximal to the origins of septal and diagonal branches are expected to produce perfusion defects in all three segments; however,

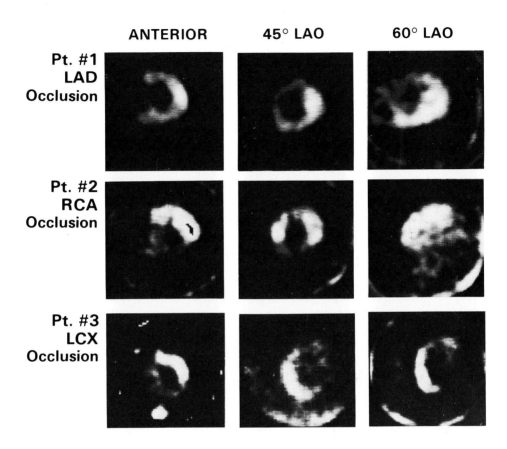

Figure 5-2. Correlation of computer processed ^{201}Tl images (anterior, 45° and 60° LAO views) in three patients with single vessel occlusions. Note the distribution of perfusion abnormalities corresponding to each vessel in different views.

distal LAD lesions should produce only apical defects. The inferior and posteroinferior segments are supplied by a dominant RCA or a dominant LCX. The posterolateral segment is supplied by marginal branches of LCX vessel. It should be pointed out that there is an overlap of distribution between different coronary arteries in some segments. For example, the diagonal branches of LAD and the marginal branches of LCX supply the lower portion of anterolateral segment as seen in the anterior view. The marginal branches of LCX and PDA may also supply the apical segment, in addition to LAD which remains the predominant source of blood supply to the apex. The 45° LAO view is the single most valuable view in the localization of perfusion defects because there is less overlap of the three segments and their respective coronary arteries.

Perfusion in Normal Heart

Monovalent cations such as thallium-201 (^{201} Tl) characteristically disappear from the blood very rapidly after an intravenous injection. The ^{201} Tl is distributed in the heart, lungs, liver and kidneys. Strauss et al. have demonstrated that myocardial uptake of ^{201} Tl correlates with regional perfusion.[5] Viable cells must also be present in these organs. The appearance of ^{201} Tl perfusion images in the normal heart has been described by Cook et al.[6] Resting thallium myocardial perfusion images display a more or less homogeneous activity in the left ventricular wall which appears as a horseshoe or ovoid pattern. The central area of relatively low activity in each view represents the left ventricular cavity.

Anterior View

In this view, the left ventricular anterolateral wall, apex and inferoposterior wall are well seen. The septal musculature is only seen occasionally. The anterolateral and inferoposterior musculature extends like two arches starting from the base of the heart and meeting as a tapering zone at the apex. The apex in some subjects is seen as a thin band (generally less than 2 cm) of low activity. Right ventricular musculature on a resting ^{201} Tl image is seen only in the presence of dilatation or hypertrophy of that chamber.

Left Anterior Oblique (LAO) Views

In the 45° view, the septal, inferior (apical) and posterolateral segments form a continuous band of uniform activity. The septal and posterolateral walls extend upward towards the mitral and aortic valve region. The septal segment generally tapers slightly near the aortic ring. In the LAO 60° view for most subjects, the apical and inferior segments are seen as separate from each other. The apex continues upward as an anteroseptal segment and inferior wall blends with posterolateral segment.

When the ^{201} Tl myocardial perfusion study is performed immediately following exercise, the overall pattern of ^{201} Tl images remains the same as described above, but with the following differences: (a) less pulmonary and splanchnic activity, (b) slight increase in myocardial activity and (c) better visualization of right ventricular myocardium.

Coronary Artery Disease

In the presence of significant coronary obstructions the regional blood flow is compromised—especially during stress, resulting in transient myocardial ischemia. The site of ischemia as well as scar from previous myocardial infarction, will show lower concentration of radioisotopes than the surrounding normal regions and are called "cold" spots on the [201] Tl images. Occasionally [201] Tl may redistribute after several hours at rest into regions where perfusion defects were shown immediately after exercise. Thus, the stress-induced ischemia can be differentiated from old myocardial infarction in most patients, because the perfusion defects produced by scar or infarction persist on the delayed images.[7] Further details of redistribution of [201] Tl on sequential imaging are discussed in Chapter 7.

As illustrated in Figures 5-2 and 5-3, it is usually possible to predict obstruction in the major coronary arteries in patients with single and double vessel coronary artery disease on the basis of [201] Tl myocardial

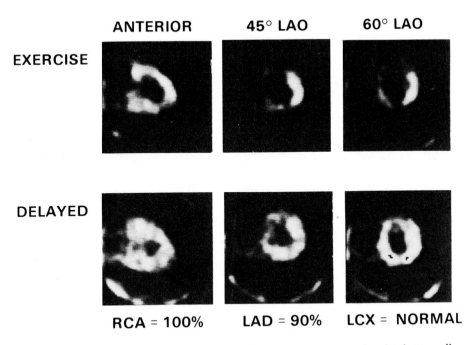

Figure 5-3.   [201]Tl images (computer processed) demonstrating septal and inferior wall ischemia in a patient with double vessel (RCA and LAD) coronary artery disease. Exercise study shows perfusion defects in the septal and inferior segments (45° to 60° LAO views). These perfusion defects improve in a 4-hour delayed study.

perfusion images. In studying comparative accuracy of [201] Tl images and the coronary angiograms of 37 male patients it was found that the sensitivity of [201] Tl imaging was good for detecting significant stenosis (>70 percent) of LAD and RCA but was poor for LCX. The overall accuracy for detection of stenosis was best for RCA (93 percent), followed by LAD (89 percent), and LCX (50 percent).[8] Lenaers et al.[2] also reported similar sensitivity and specificity for detecting disease in the individual coronary arteries. The limitation in the detection of transient ischemia in the LCX vascular region has also been shown by McLaughlin et al.[9]

A comparison of the anterior, LAO 45° and 60° views was also performed to evaluate their sensitivity to detect LAD and RCA disease. Of the 19 patients with angiographically determined LAD stenosis, hypoperfusion in the LAD region was detected from the 45° LAO view in 17 patients, but only in eight patients from either the anterior or LAO 60° views. There were 14 patients with significant RCA stenoses and of these, 13 of them demonstrated perfusion defects in the 45° LAO view and ten patients and nine patients in the anterior and LAO 60° view, respectively. Thus the 45° LAO view seems to be the best view for identifying diminished segmental perfusion in the distribution of LAD and RCA.

Limitations of [201] Tl Imaging and Angiographic Coronary Anatomy Relationship

While it is possible to predict the diseased coronary arteries from the [201] Tl images of most patients, several notable situations preclude good correlation between the segmental changes of ischemia/infarction on [201] Tl images and specific lesions in the individual coronary arteries.

Level of Exercise

If the level of exercise is not sufficient when [201] Tl is administered, either because of lack of patient motivation or associated non-cardiac disease such as peripheral vascular disease, ischemia may not result. Hence, the [201] Tl images are likely to be normal despite the presence of significant coronary lesions.

Triple Vessel Coronary Artery Disease (CAD)

The imaging technique generally underestimates the extent of myocardial ischemia or the number of diseased vessels for the following reasons: the interpretation of [201] Tl images depends on determining the relative isotope activity in different segments of the left ventricle. In other words, in a given patient with CAD, a region showing low activity (perfusion defects) is assessed in comparison to a region showing normal activity. Thus, in a patient with significant stenoses of three major coronary arteries, the region perfused by the least stenotic artery will show the greatest relative activity. Alternatively, the level of exercise at the termination of the stress test may not be sufficient to induce ischemia in the distribution of this least stenotic artery. In either case this region will be misinterpreted as normal, even though the vessel supplying it has a significant lesion. [201] Tl imaging, therefore, identifies regions with severe grades of ischemia at a given level of exercise rather than predicting the number of affected vessels. In an occasional patient with an almost equal degree of stenoses of all three major coronary arteries, the isotope activity will be uniformly reduced in all the segments, leading to an erroneous diagnosis of a normal perfusion study (Fig. 5-4). The difficulty in distinguishing the patient with double and triple vessel disease has also been reported by Lenaers et al.[2]

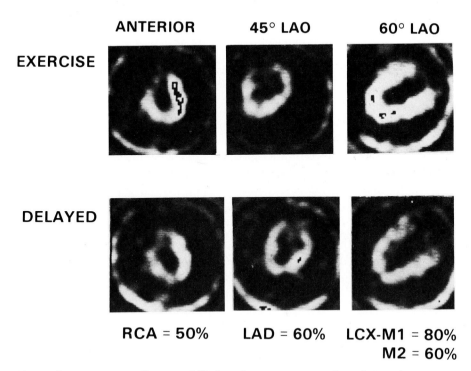

ANTERIOR   **45° LAO**   **60° LAO**

EXERCISE

DELAYED

RCA = 50%   **LAD = 60%**   **LCX-M1 = 80%**
M2 = 60%

Figure 5-4.   An essentially normal ^{201}Tl study in a patient with triple vessel coronary artery disease (see text for explanation.)

Left Main Coronary Artery (LMCA) Disease

High grade stenosis of LMCA has a serious prognosis and therefore the detection of this lesion by noninvasive means would be helpful. However, LMCA is commonly associated with additional stenoses of LAD and/or LCX arteries. As such, the presence of these additional sites of obstruction distal to the LMCA in these branches affects the location of perfusion defects and makes it almost impossible to predict the disease of the LMCA.

Variability of the Coronary Anatomy

Because the coronary artery branches vary in number and distribution, especially in the LCX and RCA systems, the assignment of perfusion defects to the respective coronary arteries is sometimes difficult. Since the RCA is dominant in 85 percent of patients, perfusion defects in the inferior segment are generally assigned to RCA lesions. However, in a significant number of patients (10 to 15 percent) perfusion defects in the inferior segment may be due to LCX disease. The contribution of an abundant collateral supply to the perfusion of a specific region of the myocardium may be another source of error in making these correlations.

Size and Location of Myocardial Lesions

Several experimental groups have shown that lesions less than one half the thickness of left ventricular wall and full-thickness lesions of less than 2.5 cm in size cannot be identified on instruments currently available.[10] Hence, a significant number of subendocardial or small transmural infarcts are missed on [201] Tl scans.

Finally, since the interpretation of [201] Tl images and coronary angiography is based on subjective parameters the role of inter- and intra-observer variability in decision making should be kept in mind. Standardized quantitative methods for the analysis of [201] Tl images have been developed to overcome some of these limitations; however, such methods are still in early stages of development.[11]

References

1. Ritchie, J.L., Trobaugh, G.B., Hamilton, G.W., et al.:   Myocardial imaging with thallium-201 at rest and during exercise: Comparison with coronary arteriography and resting and stress electrocardiography. *Circulation* **56**:66-71, 1977.

2. Lenaers, A., Black, P., van Thiel, E., et al.:   Segmental analysis of Tl-201 stress myocardial scintigraphy. *J Nucl Med* **18**:509-516, 1977.

3. James, T.N.: *Anatomy of the Coronary Arteries.* New York, Hoeber Medical Division, Harper and Row, 1961.

4. Fulton, W.F.M.: *The Coronary Arteries.* Springfield, Ill., Charles C. Thomas, 1965.

5. Strauss, H.W., Harrison, K., Langan, J.K., et al.: Thallium-201 for myocardial imaging. Relationship of thallium-201 to regional myocardial perfusion.*Circulation* **51**:641-645, 1975.

6. Cook, D.J., Bailey, I., Strauss, H.W., et al.: Thallium-201 myocardial imaging: Appearance of the normal heart. *J Nucl Med* **17**:583-589, 1976.

7. Pohost, G.M., Zir, L.M., Moore, R.H., et al.: Differentiation of transiently ischemic from infarcted myocardium by serial imaging after a single dose of thallium-201. *Circulation* **55**:294-302, 1977.

8. Bamrah, V.S., Meade, R.C., Millman, W.L., et al.: Noninvasive detection and localization of regional myocardial ischemia and infarction with thallium-201. *Clin Research* **26**:217A, 1978.

9. McLaughlin, P.R., Martin, R.P., Doherty, P., et al.: Reproducibility of thallium-201 myocardial imaging. *Circulation* **55**:497-503, 1977.

10. Strauss, H.W., and Pitt, B.: Thallium-201 as a myocardial imaging agent. *Sem Nucl Med* **7**:49, 1977.

11. Meade, R.C., Bamrah, V.S., Horgan, J.D., et al.: Quantitative methods in the evaluation of thallium-201 myocardial perfusion images. *J Nucl Med* **19**:1175-1178, 1978.

Chapter VI

Pathophysiological Basis For Abnormal Perfusion And Contraction In Coronary Artery Disease

Harold L. Brooks, M.D., and Richard Gorlin, M.D.

Our current knowledge of the pathophysiologic consequences of impaired blood flow to the myocardium is the result of scientific inquiry which began over three hundred years ago but which has become clearly focused only within the last four decades. Radionuclide techniques involving microspheres, infarct-avid agents, diffusible tracers, superior imaging instruments, minicomputers, and microprocessors have all improved our understanding of the relationship between altered contraction and regional blood flow. An understanding of the basic relationship between contraction and flow and their underlying control systems has allowed us to improve the evaluation and management of the patient with ischemic heart disease. However, we still know little about the long-term adaptive responses of the ventricle to progressive, obstructive, coronary disease. No doubt nuclear techniques will play a major role in our research within the next decade.

Anatomic Aspects of Myocardial Perfusion

We think of the coronary circulation as comprising three anatomic components: the larger epicardial vessels, the smaller resistance vessels within the myocardium, and the interarterial anastomotic channels or collaterals.

Large Epicardial Vessels

Earlier in this book (Chapter 5) Bamrah et al. present a detailed description of the normal coronary anatomy. Much of this data has come from the highly detailed anatomic injection-corrosion studies done by Fulton and James on hundreds of normal hearts during autopsy. Normally the coronary vessels are widely patent, smooth-walled and widely distributed over the epicardial surface of the heart. Nomenclature of these vessels is fairly standard. They are readily visible by coronary arteriography, and range in diameter from 10 mm in a large left main coronary artery down to 1 mm or less as they begin to penetrate the ventricular wall.

Small Resistance Vessels

These small vessels traverse the myocardium and are widely distributed from epicardial to endocardial surface. They are usually less than 1 mm in diameter and are not readily seen by routine coronary arteriography except as diffuse "myocardial blush" during late filming. They are under dynamic control of the autonomic nervous system as well as local humoral and hydraulic factors within the contracting myocardium. They are of two anatomic types: those with non-penetrating branches supply the outer and midwall layers termed Type A branches by Estes.[1] The other, more penetrating branches, traverse the entire thickness of the ventricular wall of the heart with little branching and form a subendocardial network called Type B branches. A section of the vasculature of the left ventricular wall in Figure 6-1 shows the transmural vessels forming an extensive endocardial network. Figure 6-2 shows this system schematically.[2] Because of the continual neural, humoral,and hydraulic forces acting upon these vessels there is a net dynamic resistance to flow which normally remains relatively stable, but which can change from moment to moment.

Interarterial Anastomoses

Normally interarterial anastomotic channels exist which lie dormant until obstruction or disease intervenes.[3] Microscopically these vessels appear to be derivatives of widened arterioles which are composed of an intimal lining with only a small number of surrounding medial smooth muscle cells. Little is known about how these vessels became patent and hence functional. Their significance will be discussed later in this chaper.

Physiologic Control and Reserve Systems

The experimental basis for a complex intrinsic coronary control system

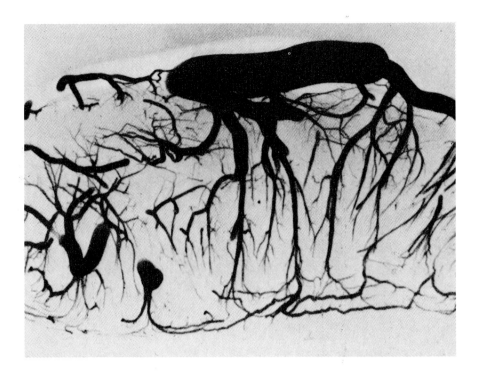

Figure 6-1. Subendocardial plexus of the left ventricle and epicardial communications through a section of left ventricular free wall. Note large epicardial artery (top). Clear demonstration of intramyocardial vessels penetrating throughout the wall and spreading into a rich endocardial network (below). (Reproduced from Fulton, W.F.M.: *The Coronary Arteries.* Springfield, Ill., Charles C. Thomas, Publishers, 1965, p. 95. Used with permission.)

is now well founded both in the experimental animal and in man. The perfusion pressures in the aorta and large coronary artery provides the driving force that delivers blood to the myocardium. Other factors that exert major influences upon the blood supply at the cellular level are epicardial/endocardial flow gradients, resistance through the small vessel network, and the arteriovenous oxygen difference. Left ventricular volume and pressure, wall tension, heart rate, and contractility all exert demands on the myocardium for available oxygen supply (Fig. 6-3). Normally the supply far exceeds the demand with a reserve capacity of three to four times resting levels.

There are four important phenomena which should be appreciated in attempting to understand perfusion of the myocardium, and the normal as well as abnormal responses that may occur.

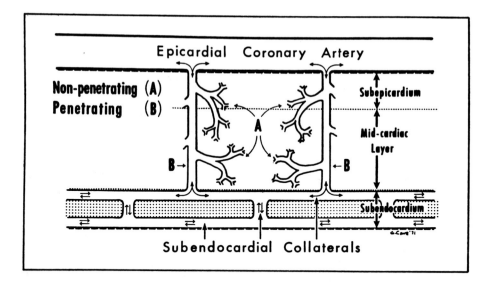

Figure 6-2. Schematic diagram of normal intramyocardial blood flow in humans. A = nonpenetrating coronary artery (Type A). B = penetrating coronary artery (Type B). Arrows demonstrate real and potential collateral flow. (Reproduced from Elliot, R. S., and Holsinger, J. W.: The pathophysiologic panorama of myocardial ischemia and infarction. In Myocardial Infarction: A new look at an old subject. Adv Cardiol, Vol. 9. Basel, S. Karger; 1973, pp. 2-15. (Used with permission.)

Coronary Blood Flow—Largely a Diastolic Phenomenon

Electromagnetic flow probes placed around the large epicardial arteries in both the experimental animal and in patients undergoing coronary surgery have shown that approximately 75 percent of blood flow occurs during diastole.[4] This is primarily because systolic wall tension starts with ventricular electrical activation spreading as a wave from the endocardium to the epicardium (Fig. 6-4). Blood flow during early and midsystole is greatly impeded, and may actually reverse itself very briefly at one point during early systole. Some blood flow does occur during late systole, however, accounting for approximately 20 to 25 percent of total coronary flow. As the wall relaxes in late systole and throughout diastole, coronary flow reaches its peak and is suddenly curtailed again at the beginning of ventricular contraction.

Coronary Autoregulation

Although the driving pressure in the aorta and large coronary arteries is

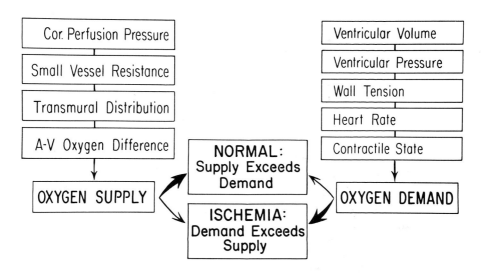

Figure 6-3. Multiple factors involved in the balance between oxygen supply (left) and oxygen demand (right).

a major determinant of blood flow to the myocardium, the ultimate delivery of blood depends heavily on both small vessel resistance and local demands regardless of perfusion pressure. There are certain limits to this autoregulatory system as illustrated by the sigmoid curve in Figure 6-5. It can be seen that over the fairly wide range from 60 to 120 mm Hg, major changes in perfusion pressure cause little change in blood flow. However, either above or below this normal physiologic range coronary flow is primarily dependent upon perfusion pressure. Autoregulatory control is mediated primarily by the resistance vessels in response to local humoral factors. The oxygen difference across the myocardium is the highest of any tissue in the body and as a result coronary venous pO_2 and presumably myocardial pO_2 are in the range of about 20 mm Hg or less. Hence myocardial oxygen extraction is near maximal levels under resting conditions.

This exquisite regulation of arteriolar resistance occurs primarily at the local level, although both alpha- and beta-adrenergic and cholinergic receptors have been demonstrated in the coronary arteries. The myocardial cell functioning at low oxygen tension can be rapidly depleted of its local oxygen supply by the slightest negative balance in the activity of the myocardial cell. This depletion results in a rapid breakdown of high energy phosphates. In the presence of a low oxygen environment, the high energy phosphates degrade by reduction and finally stabilize in the

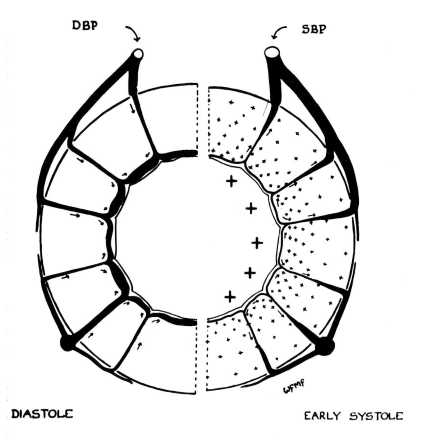

Figure 6-4. Section of left ventricle during diastole (left) and early systole (right.) (+)'s indicate increased tension at endocardium with transient reversal of blood flow (arrows) towards epicardium. (Reproduced from Fulton, W.F.M.: *The Coronary Arteries.* Springfield, Ill., Charles C. Thomas, Publishers, 1965, p. 123. Used with permission.)

form of adenosine which is freely diffusible across the cell membrane (Fig. 6-6). Being a highly potent vasodilator of the adjacent arterioles, adenosine rapidly effects immediate changes in local vascular flow in response to metabolic demands.[5]

Regional Contractile and Flow Response to Temporary Ischemia and Reflow

In the experimental animal, resting coronary blood flow is significantly altered only after stenosis has reached 80 percent.[6] Characteristically the normal myocardium responds to temporary coronary artery occlusion by an immediate diminution of contraction followed by

CORONARY AUTOREGULATION

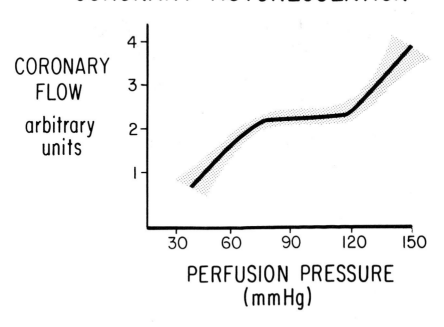

Figure 6-5. Sigmoid curve relating coronary perfusion pressure throughout the abnormal and physiologic ranges. (Reproduced from Mosher, P.: Control of coronary blood flow by an autoregulatory mechanism. *Circ Res* **14**:250-259, 1964. Used with permission of the American Heart Association, Inc.)

a prompt hypercontractile and hyperemic reaction upon release of the occlusion (Fig. 6-7).[7] The latter is essentially a "payback" phenomenon which allows an ischemic region to be replenished with oxygen following a brief ischemic episode. Other studies in animals have shown that the "payback" characteristically provides more than enough oxygen to pay the debt, and further that "payback" is directly proportional to the length of the occlusion.[4] However, if high grade stenosis is present in the artery, the payback capability is severely restricted and it is possible experimentally to totally obliterate the hyperemic response with high grade arterial stenosis.[6]

Transmural Flow Gradients

Recent experimental work by many investigators has shown that in normal dogs a significant flow gradient may readily occur between the inner and outer layers of the ventricular wall under conditions of stress

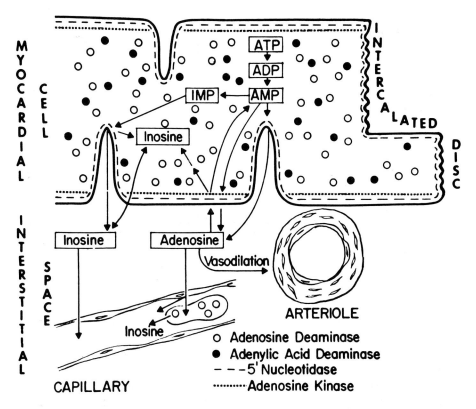

Figure 6-6. Schematic diagram of proposed pathways for synthesis, degradation, and site of action of adenosine deriving from breakdown of intracellular adenosine triphosphate. (Reproduced from Rubio, R. and Berne, R.M.: Release of adenosine by the normal myocardium in dogs and its relationship of regulation of coronary resistance. *Circ Res* **25**:407-415, 1969. Used with permission of the American Heart Association, Inc.)

where there is a competition for limited blood supply. The endocardium appears to be more vulnerable to alterations in flow and becomes ischemic more readily than does the epicardium.[8] Further experiemnts[9] have shown dramatic evidence that an ischemic layer of myocardium extends throughout the entire subendocardium as the coronary perfusion pressure is experimentally and sequentially lowered beyond physiologic levels (Fig. 6-8). The primary factors responsible for this phenomenon are greater tension in the inner half of the myocardium during systole, and distole, and increased resistance to flow through the longer Type B vessels as they penetrate the inner layers of the myocardium. Anatomic studies by Fulton[10] have shown a predominance of anastomotic connections in the endocardium which might compensate for these factors

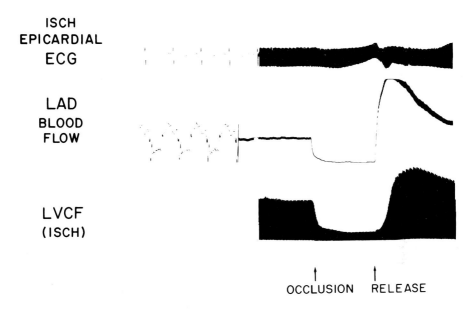

ISCH
EPICARDIAL
ECG

LAD
BLOOD
FLOW

LVCF
(ISCH)

OCCLUSION   RELEASE

Figure 6-7. Direct recordings from epicardial electrogram (ECG), left anterior descending artery (LAD) blood flow probe, and myocardial contractile force (LVCF) in an experimental animal showing the close relationship between changes in regional contraction and flow normally occurring during a brief coronary artery occlusion. The dramatic overshoot in coronary flow is characteristic and directly proportional to the length of occlusion. (Reproduced from Lichtig, C., and Brooks, H.L.: Myocardial ultrastructure and contraction during short periods of experimental ischemia. In *Recent Advances in Studies on Cardiac Structure and Metabolism*, Vol. 6. Baltimore, University Park Press, 1975. Used with permission.)

under normal conditions, but with obstructive or other diseases causing lowered perfusion pressure subendocardial ischemia may supervene, as discussed below.

Pathophysiologic Alterations in Coronary Disease

The myocardium undergoes a series of alterations during the course of obstructive coronary disease. Some are well established and predictable while others are more complex and less well understood. Coronary arteriography and radionuclide perfusion studies have greatly expanded our knowledge in this area. The interested reader is referred to a more extensive review of the entire pathophysiologic spectrum of coronary disease previously published.[11]

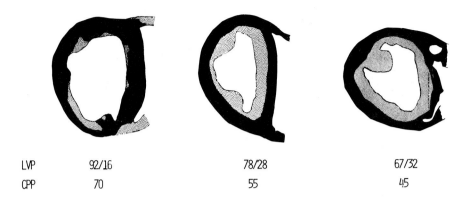

LVP	92/16	78/28	67/32
CPP	70	55	45

Figure 6-8. Experimental demonstration of a widening zone of endocardial ischemia with progressive drop in left ventricular pressure (LVP) and coronary perfusion pressure (CPP), ranging from mild deficit in CPP (70 mm Hg) and patchy mild subendocardial ischemia (left panel) to severe hypotension (CPP = 45 mm Hg) and diffuse ischemia throughout the inner half of the myocardium. (Reproduced from Salisbury, P.F., et al.: Acute ischemia of inner layers of ventricular wall. *Am Heart J* **66**:650-656, 1963. Used with permission.)

Anatomic Distribution of Coronary Disease

Coronary arteriography and postmortem studies both confirm that coronary atherosclerosis characteristically affects one or more of the proximal coronary arteries. When these arteries become critically narrowed, regional blood flow is disturbed resulting in contractile and perfusion abnormalities. Certain areas have a higher predilection for disease apparently due to hydraulic factors such as bifurcations and other areas of potential turbulence (Fig. 6-9). The major curves of the right coronary artery and left circumflex arteries are particularly prone to atheromatous lesions.[12] Major bifurcations such as the point where the left main coronary artery divides into its two branches, and the point where the artery divides into the first diagonal and first septal branches are uncommonly susceptible sites. Conversely, certain areas seem to be spared, such as the segments just beyond major bifurcations. It is frequently noted that if the marginal branches of the circumflex artery system are straight and single, they are often free of visible obstructions; but if they branch early, these sites of branching will also show evidence of disease at the tertiary branch bifurcations. Accordingly, common areas of myocardial ischemia and infarction occur in the distribution of these

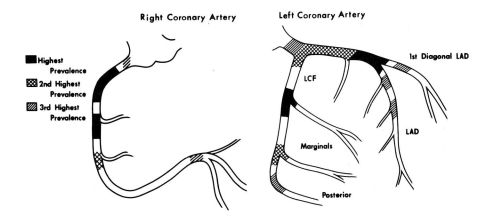

Figure 6-9. Zones of predilection of atherosclerotic lesions in the left and right coronary arteries. LAD = left anterior descending artery. LCF = left circumflex artery. (Reproduced from Gorlin, R.: *Coronary Artery Disease*. Philidelphia, W.B. Saunders Co., 1976. Used with permission.)

frequently obstructed vessels: anteroseptal, anterolateral, and inferior segments of the heart.

Collateral Circulation

Coronary collaterals no doubt play an important role in modifying myocardial perfusion defects and are probably enlargements of the normal, pre-existing interarterial anastomoses described above. There are three anatomic types of collateral pathways: epicardial, intramyocardial, and subendocardial.[13] Epicardial collaterals often take advantage of pre-existing epicardial vessels as when homolateral collaterals bypass a total obstruction in a given vessel. Intramyocardial collaterals use arteriolar connections between the distal branches of the several systems, and not infrequently the interventricular septum serves as a major pathway between right and left systems. The subendocardial plexus may provide another intramyocardial bypass around an obstruction when the perforating blood vessels anastomose with the subendocardial plexus to form a bridge around the obstruction.

The nature, purpose, and control of these vascular connections have been the subject of controversy in the literature for many years. While the actual mechanism for becoming patent and functional is not well understood, a pressure difference between two adjacent vascular beds and local tissue hypoxia seem to be major factors.

It is most likely that the initiating event is a significant pressure difference between two adjacent vascular beds. This persistant pressure gradient opens up dormant interarterial anastomotic channels.[14] Evidence from acute occlusions of coronary arteries in dogs indicates that collateral flow will occur rapidly from a neighboring coronary vessel. The more distal the applied obstruction, the greater the likelihood of retrograde flow. Collateral vessels are not seen when obstruction is less than 50 percent of the lumen of the major artery.[15] Thus, collaterals seem to function only when there is severe obstruction of the coronary artery generating a low distal pressure in one part of the system. However, this is not always the rule since collateral vessels do not form in 15 to 20 percent of patients with major obstructing lesions.[16] Several reasons may account for this: (a) The portion of myocardium being served by the vessel is no longer functioning as active myocardium. (b) The muscle may be deriving its blood supply from vascular roots not visualized by usual techniques (e.g., extracoronary collaterals from pericardial or bronchial arteries). (c) The given arterial obstruction may be so situated that the distal coronary artery cannot be supplied from a neighboring coronary artery because it too is obstructed and perfusion pressure is no higher than in the first artery. Under such circumstances the hydraulic potential for collateral flow is compromised and in fact, such a circumstance may lead to the phenomenon of coronary "steal," when certain areas of the myocardium are perfused at the expense of others.[8]

The Wide Spectrum of Perfusion and Contractile Abnormalities

While coronary disease is considered to be segmental in distribution, it may in fact be global, or exhibit manifestations anywhere between these two extremes. Accordingly, contractile and perfusion dysfunction can be global or segmental, subendocardial or transmural, depending upon the distribution of the underlying disease process. Terminology proposed by Herman et al. [17] has been widely accepted and proven helpful in describing specific abnormal contractile patterns (Fig. 6-10). Segmental contractile dysfunction or asynergy occurs more frequently than global dysfunction and generalized hypokinesis. Likewise, localized perfusion defects are probably more common than generalized or global hypoperfusion although the latter is difficult to assess in patients since present clinical methods depend upon relative rather than absolute flow levels.

Acute myocardial necrosis usually causes fibrocollagenous scar. The scar may take on a number of different forms, the commonest being the intramyocardial scar, formed in a plaque-like distribution along the inner third of the heart wall. This type of subendocardial necrosis usually

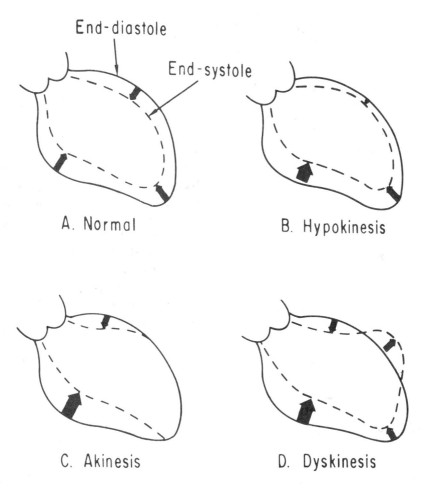

Figure 6-10. Localized and generalized abnormalities in cardiac contraction showing end-diastole and end-systole superimposed and excursion represented by arrows. (Reproduced from Herman, M.V., et al.: Localized disorders in myocardial contraction: Asynergy and its role in congestive heart failure. *N Engl J Med* **277**:222-232, 1967. Used with permission.)

occurs without frank occlusion of pre-existing narrowed coronary arteries. The other obvious form of damage is the full-thickness scar which follows transmural myocardial infarction. This type of infarction is now considered to be a consequence of acute occlusion—usually thrombosis of the nutrient coronary artery.[18]

There are specific pathologic conditions which can compromise intramyocardial or subendocardial perfusion even when there is no thrombosis or occlusion of major vessels. The subendocardium of the left ventricle is particularly susceptible to perfusion abnormalities not solely because of its dependence upon the longer (and thus higher resistance) Type B vessels, but because of the higher intramyocardial wall tension. During systole the myocardial tension and resultant compression and distortion of the perforating vessels limit the effectiveness of systolic perfusion. Tension within the wall of the myocardium is highest at the endocardial rim and progressively decreases toward the epicardial surface. Hence there is a progressive resistance to perfusion from the epicardium to the endocardium during systole. Intramyocardial tension can also be affected during the diastolic phase of the cardiac cycle, and this pressure can be no lower than the tension due to intracavitary diastolic pressure. During ischemia, end-diastolic pressure rises, as the wall of the myocardium stiffens during diastole, and consequently impedance to flow increases in the subendocardial layer resulting in loss of collateral channels within the subendocardial network. If the damage is small, ischemia may remain circumscribed with relatively limited eventual scar. On the other hand, a large ischemic area in the anterior and septal myocardium may result in more widespread hemodynamic changes. If cardiac failure occurs and left ventricular diastolic pressure rises, further increase in endocardial tension supervenes and the resistance in the subendocardial network rises even higher. This has been termed the "hemodynamic vise" of the subendocardium, (Fig. 6-11),[2] and may produce a vicious cycle of intractable heart failure.

Perfusion and Contractile Abnormalities Induced During Stress

It has now been amply demonstrated that induced stress can produce both contractile and perfusion abnormalities not demonstrable during the resting state. Several maneuvers have been successfully used to produce adequate stress levels in patients: (a) supine bicycle ergometer exercise, (b) isoproterenol infusion, (c) rapid volume infusion, (d) atrial pacing, and (e) sustained hand grip.

All five methods of stress can impose increased oxygen demands upon the heart—albeit to varying degrees. Controlled supine bicycle exercise produces the most physiologic effect that can be conveniently applied in the laboratory and has been used frequently in cardiac catheterization studies and, more recently, in noninvasive radionuclide studies. During physical exercise, there is increased vasomotor activity, blood is returned to the heart resulting in augmentation of the Starling Effect. Concurrently, sympathetic nerves are stimulated causing an increase in rate-augmented inotropic state, and reduced impedance to ejection by peripheral vasodilation. Thus physical exercise is associated with a generalized peripheral effect as well as increased central cardiac inotropic

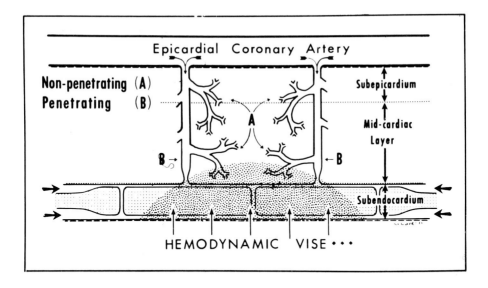

Figure 6-11. Schematic diagram of intramyocardial blood flow in subendocardial ischemia illustrating "hemodynamic vise" restricting blood flow in deep endocardial layers.
(Reproduced from Eliot, R.S., and Holsinger, J.W.: The pathophysiologic panorama of
myocardial ischemia and infarction. In Myocardial Infarction: A new look at an old subject. Adv. Cardiol. Vol. 9. Basel, S. Karger, 1973, pp. 2-15. Used with permission.)

and chronotropic activity. These alterations of myocardial mechanical
activity increase oxygen consumption and lead to an increase in myocardial blood flow. This is depicted in Figure 6-12 where myocardial
oxygen consumption increases in response to stress. The normal heart
can meet the demand by a virtually linear increase in coronary blood
flow. In the presence of disease, the myocardial segment is served by
a critically obstructed coronary artery, myocardial blood flow cannot
respond to meet the energy demand and this abnormality appears on the
radionuclide scan as a poorly perfused area of the myocardium, or on the
gated blood pool study as a contraction abnormality. Normally auto-
regulation would lead to a dilatation of coronary arterioles. However,
arteriolar vasodilation in postobstructed segments is usually already
maximal to compensate for deficits in perfusion pressure resulting from
the arterial obstruction. Thus segments of myocardial vasculature may
be unable to dilate further producing a heterogeneity in regional blood
flow and a difference in the absolute quantity of radionuclide available
for exchange in different myocardial capillary beds.

Another important factor in the pathophysiology of perfusion defects is
that the transmembrane distribution of cations depends upon intact
cell-membrane function. As previously mentioned, adenosine triphos-

EFFECT OF INCREASED CARDIAC ENERGY DEMAND ON LOCAL BLOOD SUPPLY

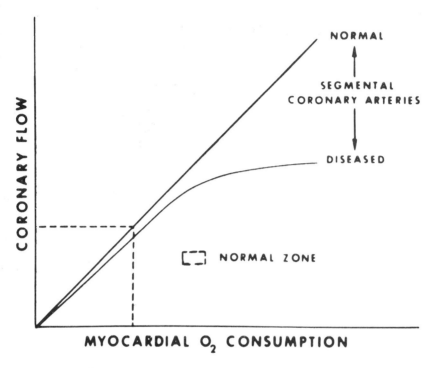

Figure 6-12. Effect of increased energy demands by the heart on local blood supply during stress showing linear relationship of coronary flow to myocardial oxygen consumption in the normal heart, and the fall-off that occurs in coronary flow during higher energy loads in the diseased hears. (Reproduced from Gorlin, R.: *Coronary Artery Disease.* Philadelphia, W.B. Saunders Co., 1976. Used with permission.)

phatase, actively maintains an optimal electrochemical gradient of potassium and sodium across the cell membrane. During myocardial ischemia induced by hypoxia and stress, there is a significant alteration in membrane enzyme function, significantly reducing the cell's ability to extract potassium and other cations including thallium-201.[19] We have illustrated elsewhere in this book examples of exercise-induced thallium perfusion defects from patients with normal resting scans. Such stress/exercise comparisons in both perfusion and contraction radionuclide studies have now been demonstrated to be powerful techniques in the assessment and follow-up of selected patients with coronary disease.

References

1. Estes, E.H., Entman, M.L., Dixon, H.B., et al.: The vascular supply of the left ventricular wall. *Am Heart J* **71**:58-67, 1966.

2. Eliot, R.S., and Holsinger, J.W.: The pathophysiologic panorama of myocardial ischemia and infarction. In Myocardial Infarction: A new look at an old subject. Adv Cardiol. Vol. 9. Basel, S. Karger. 1973, pp. 2-15.

3. Schaper, J., Borgers, M., and Schaper, W.: Ultrastructure of ischemia-induced changes in the precapillary anastomotic network of the heart. *Am J Cardiol* **29**:851-859, 1972.

4. Gregg, D.E., and Sabiston, D.C.: Current research and problems of the coronary circulation. *Circulation* **13**:916-927, 1956.

5. Rubio, R., and Berne, R.M.: Release of adenosine by the normal myocardium in dogs and its relationship of regulation of coronary resistance. *Circ Res* **25**:407-415, 1969.

6. Gould, K.L., Hamilton, G.W., Lipscomb, K., et al.: Method for assessing stress-induced regional malperfusion during coronary arteriography: Experimental validation and clinical application. *Am J Cardiol* **34**:557-564, 1974.

7. Lichtig, C., and Brooks, H.L.: Myocardial ultrastructure and contraction during short periods of experimental ischemia. In *Recent Advances in Studies on Cardiac Structure and Metabolism*, Vol. 6. Baltimore, University Park Press, 1975, p. 423.

8. Downey, J.N. and Kirk, E.S.: Distribution of the coronary blood flow across the canine heart wall during systole. *Circ Res.* **34**:251-257, 1974.

9. Salisbury, P.F., Cross, C.E., and Rieben, A.P.: Acute ischemia of inner layers of ventricular wall. *Am Heart J* **66**:650-656, 1963.

10. Fulton, W.F.M.: *The Coronary Arteries.* Springfield, Ill., Charles C. Thomas Publisher, 1965, p. 128.

11. Gorlin, R.: *Coronary Artery Disease.* Philadelphia, W.B. Saunders Co., 1976.

12. Glagov, S.: Hemodynamic risk factors: Mechanical stress, mural architecture, medial nutrition, and the vulnerability of arteries to atherosclerosis. In Wissler, R.W., and Geer, J.C. (Eds.): *The Pathogenesis of Atherosclerosis.* Baltimore, Williams and Wilkins Co., 1972.

13. Blumgart, H.L., Zoll, P.M., Freedberg, A.S., et al.: The experimental production of intercoronary anastomoses and their functional significance. *Circulation* **1**:10-27, 1950.

14. Kattus, A.A., and Gregg, D.E.: Some determinants of coronary collateral blood flow in the open-chest dog. *Circ Res* **7**:628-642, 1959.

15. Gensini, G.G., and de Costa, B.C.B.: The coronary collateral circulation in living man. *Am J Cardiol* **24**:393-400, 1969.

16. Helfant, R.H., Vokonas P.S., and Gorlin, R.: Functional importance of the human coronary collateral circulation. *N Engl J Med* **284**:1277-1281, 1971.

17. Herman, M.V., Heinle, R.A., Klein, M.D., et al.: Localized disorders in myocardial contraction: Asynergy and its role in congestive heart failures. *N Engl J Med* **277**:222-232, 1967.

18. Chandler, A.B., Chapman, I., Erhardt, L.R., et al.: Coronary thrombosis in the myocardial infarction. Report of a workshop on the role of coronary thrombosis in the pathogenesis of acute myocardial infarction. *Am J Cardiol* **34**:823-833, 1974.

19. Counsell, R.E., Yu, T., Ranode, V., et al.: Radioiodinated bretyllium analogs for myocardial scanning. *J Nucl Med* **15**:991-996, 1974.

CHAPTER VII

Thallium-201 Myocardial Redistribution for the Diagnosis of Coronary Artery Disease

Kenneth A. McKusick, M.D.
H. William Strauss, M.D.
John Bingham, M.D.
Gerald M. Pohost, M.D.
Timothy E. Guiney, M.D.

Sudden death is the initial manifestation in one-third of patients with coronary artery disease (CAD) in this country. In 1975 nearly 700,000 people died of this disease (Table 7-1). Clearly, a noninvasive procedure was needed to detect the presence of coronary artery disease in patients who are still asymptomatic.

From the mid-1930's until the early 1970's, the exercise electrocardiographic (ECG) stress test, introduced by Master, was the only nonin-

TABLE 7-1
Death Rate CAD (1975)

Age years	Per 100,000
< 34	5
44	45
54	180
64	500
74	1200
84	5000
680,000 annually	60% sudden!

Supported in Part by NIH Training Grant #1-T32-HL-07416-01.

vasive method for detecting myocardial ischemia. Myocardial perfusion imaging during exercise stress tests was introduced in the 1970's.[1] Although the exercise ECG stress test is valuable, its sensitivity ranges from 54 to 80 percent, and depends upon the ability of a patient to achieve maximum heart rate before the test is completed. Further, the specificity of an ECG stress test in asymptomatic patients is low. Less than 65 percent of patients with an abnormal ECG stress test actually have significant coronary artery disease on angiographic examination of the coronary arteries. The addition of an exercise myocardial perfusion stress test has increased the sensitivity and specificity of exercise stress testing.[2,3]

The exercise ECG stress test is frequently used to evaluate a patient with possible coronary artery disease. The likelihood of myocardial ischemia is low and no further procedure may be indicated if, in the presence of a normal blood pressure response and high heart rate at peak exercise, the electrocardiogram is normal. If the results of the ECG stress test are uncertain, a thallium-201 stress test is indicated. With a normal thallium-201 exercise stress test the likelihood of coronary artery disease is less than 5 percent; whereas an abnormal thallium-201 exercise stress study raises the likelihood of myocardial ischemia to greater than 85 percent, regardless of ECG changes or symptoms during the exercise procedure.[4,5] A decision to do a coronary angiographic examination of a patient will depend upon the results of thallium-201 exercise stress test (Fig. 7-1). The decision to follow one or the other branch of a diagnostic tree is based upon the certainty of a specific test result, the reliability of the test to predict the presence or absence of disease, and the condition of the patient.

Thallium-201 exercise stress tests are noninvasive functional measurements which assess the adequacy of regional myocardial blood flow

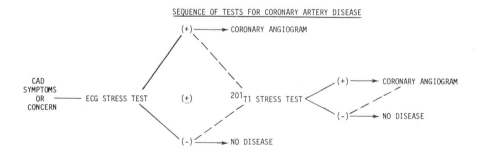

SEQUENCE OF TESTS FOR CORONARY ARTERY DISEASE

Figure 7-1.

under conditions of maximum cardiac work. The validity of the resulting measurements is reduced if a maximum work load cannot be reached. Anatomic, rather than functional measurements are determined by coronary angiography, which provides excellent spatial resolution of the coronary arteries. The adequacy of myocardial perfusion distal to a detected coronary arterial lesion, especially in response to increased cardiac work, can only be inferred from that noninvasive procedure.

Physiology

The noninvasive measurement of regional myocardial perfusion with thallium-201 is predicated on Sapirstein's principle which states that if a substance is rapidly cleared from the blood, and if that substance is concentrated in an organ, then its regional concentration is related to blood flow.[6] Thallium-201, as thallous chloride, is a monovalent cation potassium analog which is rapidly cleared from the blood by many organs of the body including the myocardium.[7-9] The total body distribution of thallium-201 reflects cardiac output to all organs except the brain, where it is normally excluded by the blood-brain barrier. After thallium is injected, it is distributed in the body and then slowly reaches equilibrium. During the first transit of thallium-201 to the coronary vascular bed, 88 percent of the tracer is extracted. The distribution of thallium-201 throughout the body is markedly different when the patient is at rest than when the patient is exercising at maximum levels, and this difference reflects cardiac output (Fig. 7-2). The profound difference is secondary to a shunting of cardiac output away from the splanchnic region to cardiac and skeletal muscles.[10] Regional differences in uptake of thallium by a normal myocardium and a myocardium perfused by a stenotic vessel may not be detected in a patient at rest. In response to increased metabolic demand, a normal coronary artery system can augment blood flow up to five times the normal basal value. The precapillary arterial sphincter of a stenotic vessel, which is already maximally dilated, cannot respond to increased metabolic demand in a similar way.[11] The thallium-201 images taken of the heart with the patient at maximum exercise will represent regional myocardial blood flow and will reflect the varying capacity of the coronary arterial bed to respond to increased metabolic needs of the myocardium. Thus, in the presence of coronary artery disease, areas where thallium-201 activity is reduced or absent represent zones of decreased perfusion. If a defect can be seen on a myocardial thallium-201 perfusion image when the tracer is injected while the patient is exercising at maximum levels, and none is

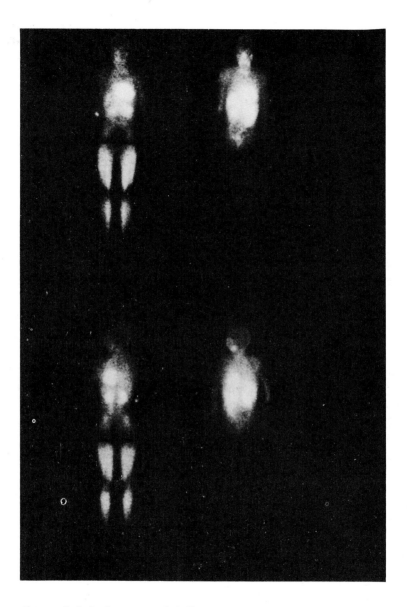

Figure 7-2.   Whole body images of thallium-201 studies done with the patient exercising (left) and at rest (right). The distribution of thallium-201 reflects cardiac output at the time thallium is injected. In addition to the marked increase in thallium activity in the cardiac and skeletal muscles of the exercising patient, there is reduced splanchnic activity which reflects a shunting of blood away from that region as exercise begins.

seen when the injection is given with the patient at rest, there is transient ischemia secondary to stenosis or spasm of the coronary artery supplying that region. A perfusion defect that is present on thallium scans taken with the patient at rest and while exercising is probably indicative of scar. The phenomenon of thallium-201 redistribution, which occurs following intravenous injection, permits imaging of a patient immediately following maximum exercise and later to provide early and late images representative of myocardial blood flow when the heart is at maximum stress and in the resting state.[12-14] In humans undergoing stress testing, myocardial thallium-201 activity is reduced over the ensuing 2.5 hours by 25 percent.

Thallium-201 is redistributed throughout the entire body following intravenous injection (Fig. 7-3). Over 95 percent of thallium-201 injected intravenously while the patient is at rest or exercising is taken up initially by tissues other than the myocardium. Thallium-201 outside the heart becomes available for redistribution over the next several hours providing thallium-201 levels in the bloodstream are low, and clear in accordance with cardiac output. Even though they are not fully understood, the kinetics of thallium-201 redistribution appears to depend on persistence of a low level of thallium in the blood and a trend toward equilibration in body tissues.

An experimental investigation into the kinetics and pharmacokinetics of thallium-201 redistribution in animals showed that in normally perfused myocardium, thallium-201 activity reaches an early maximum and slowly clears (Fig. 7-4). When a persistent, complete occlusion is applied by a snare to the left anterior descending coronary artery in dogs, a low and essentially unchanged level of thallium-201 activity is measured in the myocardial bed of the affected artery. If the occlusive snare is released after injection of thallium-201, there is a rapid accumulation of thallium-201. By maintaining a partial occlusion (stenosis) rather than a complete occlusion of the LAD, a gradual increase of activity can be observed in the myocardium distal to the partial occlusion. When partial occlusion is maintained, there is an initial reduction in the uptake of thallium, and rather than clearance as in normally perfused myocardium, a rising level of activity results. The thallium-201 activity in nonischemic and ischemic myocardium during redistribution is the result of a complex of kinetics including the concentration of thallium-201 in blood, regional myocardial blood flow, and the rates of thallium transport in and out of the intact myocardial cell.[15-17] Current experimental data indicate that concentration of thallium-201 ions seeks equilibrium between myocardium and blood, and that ischemia may affect the kinetics of cellular transport of thallium and cause a reduced clearance rate.

Thallium-201 is redistributed in the human heart in a manner similar to the experimental model. If a myocardial defect seen on thallium-201

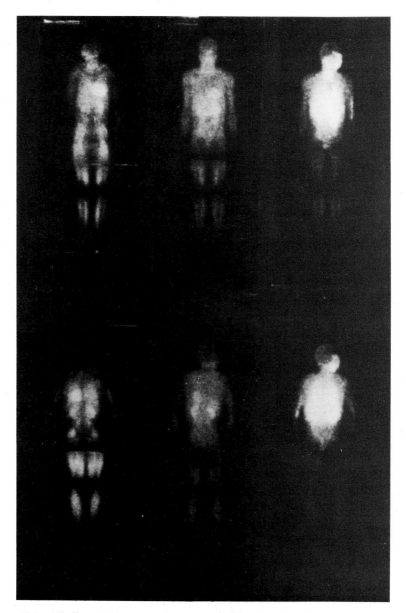

Figure 7-3. Thallium-201 scan with exercise (left) and redistribution image 24 hours later (middle), whole body images (right) injected with the patient at rest. Essentially no thallium-201 is excreted in the first 24 hours after injection. Thus, even though thallium-201 rapidly moves intracellularly following injection, a sustained low level of thallium-201 is slowly redistributed into the blood in concordance with resting cardiac output. Because of the kinetics of thallium-201 clearance from muscle, the 24-hour redistribution image more closely resembles the image of the patient injected during exercise than the image of the patient injected at rest.

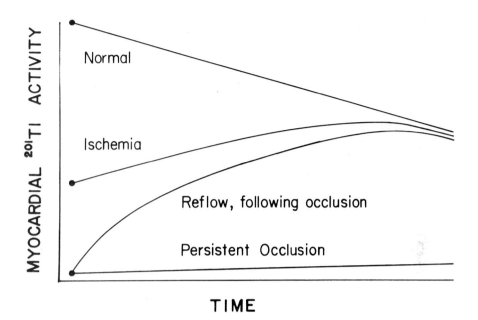

Figure 7-4. Schematic representation of thallium-201 activity in the myocardium of animals in several experimental models representative of disease in humans. A *complete occlusion* is created by a snare around the left anterior descending coronary artery. Thallium-201 activity distal to the occlusion remains low and essentially unchanged. If the snare is removed several minutes after thallium-201 is injected, flow resumes as it does after transient coronary spasm, and thallium-201 accumulates rapidly. Thallium-201 activity is reduced distal to a *partial occlusion (ischemia),* but slowly increased even though the partial LAD occlusion is maintained. Under *normal* conditions thallium-201 activity reaches an early maximum following intravenous injection and then clears from myocardium.

scan does not disappear, the presumptive diagnosis is myocardial scar. On the other hand, a defect on a myocardial perfusion scan which disappears with time can be presumed to represent coronary stenosis with associated myocardial ischemia. No data are available at present to determine how often ischemia, as measured by coronary venous lactate levels, correlates with defects induced by transient exercise and seen on thallium-201 scans.[18]

Sensitivity and Specificity

The "gold" standard by which ECG and thallium-201 stress measurements are judged is coronary angiography. Assuming that significant stenosis represents a narrowing of 50 percent or greater, the sensitivity of thallium-201 stress testing in a series of patients was 86 percent and the specificity 78 percent (Fig. 7-5). The sensitivity of the ECG stress testing by itself was 54 percent in the same population. A false abnormal thallium-201 stress test may result from several causes including mitral valve prolapse, coronary bridging, and subcritical stenosis (that is, stenosis less than 50 percent). The significance of a transient defect induced by exercise during thallium-201 scanning in the presence of a subcritical stenosis demonstrated on coronary angiography is uncertain. It is likely, however, that the coronary lesion is hemodynamically significant.

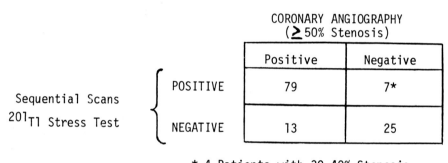

CORONARY ANGIOGRAPHY
($\geq$ 50% Stenosis)

Sequential Scans ^{201}Tl Stress Test		Positive	Negative
	POSITIVE	79	7*
	NEGATIVE	13	25

* 4 Patients with 30-40% Stenosis

Figure 7-5

The predictive value of an abnormal thallium-201 exercise stress test in this series was 92 percent. The sensitivity and specificity were both less than 90 percent.[2-4] The value of a test such as this depends in great part upon the population which is examined. It is most certainly applicable in those patients with a moderate likelihood of coronary artery disease, but should not be considered as a screening test for coronary artery disease in the population at large.

At present the major indication for a thallium-201 stress test is to improve the accuracy of the ECG exercise testing (Table 7-2). Fundamental to that precept is that all thallium-201 stress testing should be preceded by an ECG stress test, and the patients who should be referred for thallium-201 stress test are those in whom no definitive diagnosis can be made on the basis of the exercise ECG stress test alone. An example is one series of patients (Table 7-3) who had positive ECG changes, but who did not have typical chest pain in response to maximum stress. The

TABLE 7-2
Indications for Tl^{201} Stress Test

Definite:	Improve accuracy of exercise test
Relative:	Define zone of ischemia
	acute myocardial infarction
	variant or unstable angina
	S/P CABG or medical therapy

thallium-201 stress test was 89 percent sensitive and 88 percent specific for the detection of coronary artery disease in that group, with a predictive value for abnormal studies of 95 percent. Only one patient had significant coronary artery disease with a normal thallium-201 stress scan. The patient had an 80 percent stenosis of a short left anterior descending coronary artery, and the entire left ventricular apex was supplied by an unusually long posterior descending coronary artery originating from the right coronary artery.[19]

TABLE 7-3
ECG Abnormal Exercise Test: Asymptomatic Or Atypical Chest Pain

	Tl (-)	Tl (+)
CA (-)	23	3°
CA (+)	1	8

Sensitivity 89 percent: Specificity 88 percent

°2 subcritical stenosis
1 mitral valve prolapse

Many patients with atypical chest pain can be evaluated on the basis of a normal exercise ECG stress test. There are patients with atypical chest pain, who are symptomatic with normal ECG changes on stress testing, where reassurance does not suffice and further procedures such as thallium-201 can be helpful. In addition to those patients, other circumstances which make the ECG difficult to interpret, such as bundle branch block or digitalis effect, are indications for a thallium-201 exercise test (Table 7-4).

Interpretation

In some patients abnormal increased pulmonary activity has been

TABLE 7-4
Indications (Examples)

Asymptomatic patient with significant findings on annual physical examination (ECG changes, high lipids, family history).

Atypical chest pain with nondiagnostic ECG stress test.

Abnormal ECG stress test with productive atypical chest pain.

Factors effecting ECG interpretation (left bundle branch block, resting Q or ST abnormalities, hypertension, digitalis).

noted during stress testing on first images taken following injection of thallium-201 (Fig. 7-6). Usually the increased activity of thallium-201 in the lungs is seen on initial images but is not apparent on delayed images. In one series of patients without significant coronary artery disease, the heart to lung activity ratio of thallium-201 was found to be above 2:1; whereas in 78 patients with double or triple vessel coronary artery disease, the ratio fell below 2:1. It is probable that two factors account for the finding of increased pulmonary activity in patients with ischemia following exercise stress testing. One is delayed pulmonary transit time, and the second is increased left ventricular end-diastolic pressure secondary to reduced left ventricular functional reserve. Increased pulmonary activity is not pathognomonic of coronary artery disease, since diminished left ventricular functional reserve can be seen in noncoronary artery disease, including cardiomyopathy, valvular disease, or extensive myocardial scar. However, since the population undergoing exercise stress testing is primarily under evaluation for suspected coronary artery disease, increased pulmonary activity is a good indicator of impaired left ventricular function.[20] In that setting, impaired left ventricular function is usually secondary to coronary artery disease. The finding of increased concentration of thallium-201 in the lungs increases the sensitivity of thallium-201 stress imaging in patients with coronary artery disease who are unable to exercise to predicted maximum work loads. These patients may not alter regional coronary blood flow sufficiently to permit detection of coronary artery disease by thallium-201 imaging; in those patients the only manifestation of coronary artery disease may be increased pulmonary activity of thallium-201 (Fig. 7-7).

Several factors should be considered in the interpretation of a thallium stress test. A prime consideration is the adequacy of the exercise portion of the test to induce a work load on the heart sufficient to demonstrate

Ex.   Delay

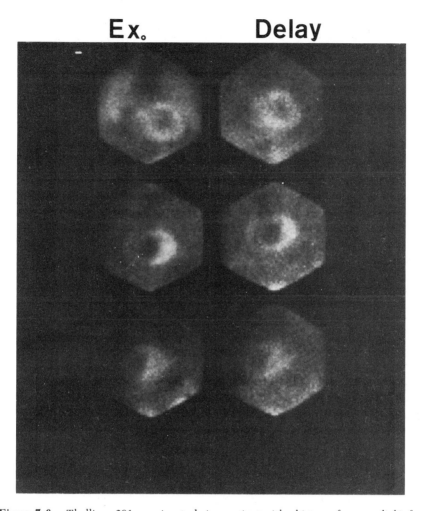

Figure 7-6. Thallium-201 exercise study in a patient with a history of myocardial infarction and triple vessel CAD. (Initial images after exercise, left; two-hour delayed images, right. Anterior, 45° LAO, 60° LAO projections from top to bottom). There is a septal defect ion the initial 45° LAO image which persists on the delayed study, and indicates a scar. No stress induced ischemia defects are seen in the myocardium. Initial anterior images show that pulmonary activity is increased moderately with stress, secondary to reduced left ventricular reserve. The patient's stress test was terminated after 4.5 minutes because of fatigue and dyspnea.

regional differences in blood flow by transient changes in activity of thallium-201 in the myocardium. Some patients, in addition to those who are unable to reach maximum effort because of coronary artery disease, may not be able to give maximal effort for other reasons, such as

Ex. Delay

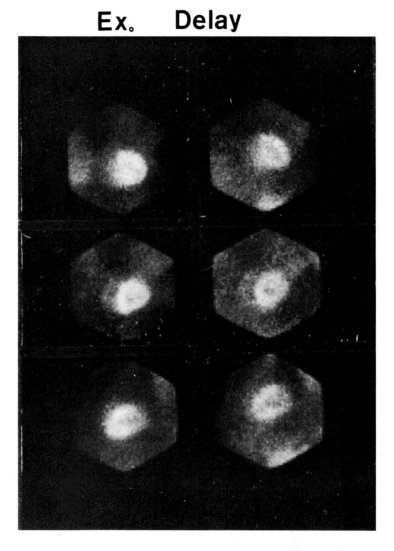

Figure 7-7. Thallium-201 exercise study in a patient with a history of angina pectoris, recently asymptomatic while on propranolol. (Initial images after exercise; left; two-hour delayed images, right. Anterior, 45° LAO, 60° LAO projections from top to bottom). Has 70% stenosis in LAD, 50% stenosis in the circumflex artery. Exercise stress test was terminated by fatigue. The ECG was normal. The thallium-201 images of the myocardial appear normal without any defects. However, initial images show moderately increased pulmonary activity, not seen on the delayed pictures. Pulmonary thallium-201 activity induced by exercise occasionally is the only finding suggestive of underlying cardiac disease.

pulmonary insufficiency or intermittent claudication. The main criteria
for judging the adequacy of an exercise test is the ability to achieve 85
percent or greater of maximum predicted heart rate. A clue to the
adequacy of exercise can also be found from review of the initial thal-
lium-201 image (Fig. 7-8, *A* and *B*). When maximum exercise has
been reached, there is no discernible thallium-201 activity in the liver.
In the presence of thallium-201 activity in the splanchnic region, it is
unlikely that the patient reached a maximum exercise level. An additional indicator of submaximal work load is the absence of right

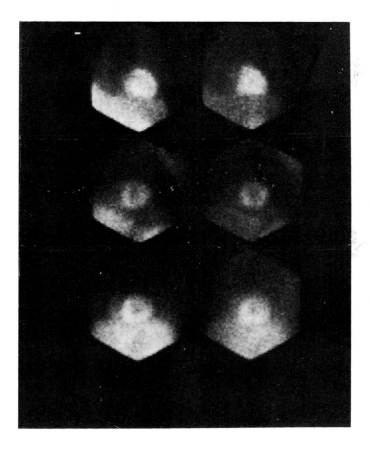

Figure 7-8A. Normal thallium-201 cardiac study injected at rest on a patient with
normal coronary artery angiogram (initial images 15 minutes after injection, left; two-
hour delayed redistribution images, right; anterior, 45° LAO, 60° LAO projections, top,
middle, bottom.) Myocardial activity is normal and appears homogeneous on thallium-
201 scans. On rest injected images, the normal right ventricle is not distinctly seen, and
hepatic activity is present.

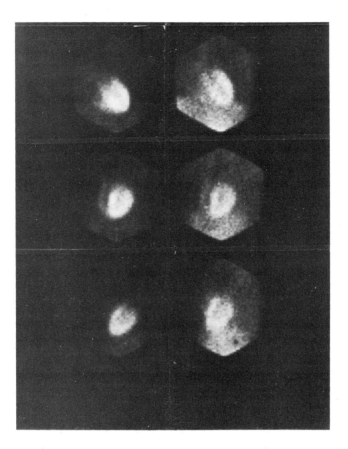

Figure 7-8B. Normal thallium-201 exercise study of a patient with normal coronary angiogram (initial images five minutes after injection, left: two-hour delayed redistribution images, right; anterior, 45° LAO, 60° LAO projections top, middle, bottom). There is homegeneous distribution of thallium-201 activity in the left ventricle, and the right ventricle is distinctly seen on the 60° LAO projection. No hepatic activity is appreciated on the initial images taken immediately after exercise. Two hours later the myocardial activity has decreased, and there has been some redistribution into the subdiaphragmatic region including the liver.

ventricular activity. Normally, the right ventricle, which is of less mass than the left ventricle, is only minimally visualized on thallium-201 scans injected with the patient at rest, but is seen following an injection during maximal exercise. When the right ventricle is not visualized on a stress study, there has either been submaximal exercise, or there is ischemia or scar of the right ventricle.[21]

The validity of a thallium stress test depends not only upon the level of exercise, but on when the initial imaging was done after the injection. Redistribution begins promptly, particularly if the degree of stenosis is not great. Images should begin no more than five minutes after injection, and the entire first set of images should be completed within the next 30 minutes. To complete this sequence on time, images recorded for 10 minutes each at the 80 keV mercury x-ray window with an all purpose collimator in anterior, 45°, and 60° anterior oblique projections provide adequate statistical data.

Image Interpretation

The interpretation of thallium-201 myocardial images can be difficult, but if one follows a format of inspection, the ambiguities are reduced (Fig. 7-9 and Table 7-5). The adequacy of the exercise test is evaluated

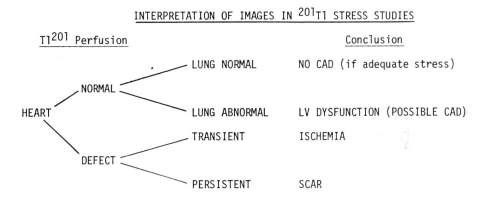

Figure 7-9.

by observation of the level of splanchnic activity on the initial image. The size and thickness of the left and right ventricles is assessed and consideration given to the possibility of cardiac disease, other than coronary artery disease, which may cause ventricular hypertrophy or dilatation. The left ventricle may be dilated immediately after exercise, as seen on the first anterior image following exercise. This appearance could be misinterpreted on delayed images as redistribution. The most difficult areas to interpret have been the high septum and posterior walls, where one is uncertain whether an absence of thallium activity is related to a valve plane or the presence of ischemia or scar. Clearly, if on

TABLE 7-5.
Considerations While Reading Tl^{201} Stress Images

Adequacy of Exercise
Lung Activity
Heart Cavity—Size (Initial and Delayed)
Myocardial Thickness
Right Ventricle
Difficult Areas—Upper Septum, Posterior Wall

delayed images a border zone fills in, then the diagnosis is ischemia (Figs. 7-10 and 7-11).

The myocardium represents an unusual problem for nuclear imaging since it is a cone which is continuously moving in the relatively lengthy process of imaging. Gating of the scintillation camera can be useful to eliminate some of the blurring caused by cardiac motion, particularly if images are recorded throughout the entire diastolic interval. However, even with the gating technique, contrast between myocardium and background is limited. The viewer can see alterations in myocardial perfusion more readily if the thallium images are displayed on a computer so that contrast may be enhanced. Contrast enhancement is a two-edged sword, since the myocardium normally has some heterogeneity of flow and the number of counts in an area of myocardium may fluctuate by as much as 14 percent. These factors cause images that have a mottled appearance, and which may be difficult to interpret. Smoothing the data by digital averaging techniques, or simply by squinting at the image does help reduce some of the problems. Phantom studies have demonstrated that lesions less than one-half the full thickness of the myocardium and smaller than 2.5 cm in diameter, or less than 5 grams in mass may not be delineated. Further studies with phantoms suggest that a reduction of activity of greater than 25 percent to an area of at least 2.5 cm is required for visualization of a lesion with thallium-201 myocardial imaging.

Most laboratories which perform thallium-201 exercise stress tests take initial stress images and then redistribution serial images to differentiate viable, though ischemic myocardium from regions of myocardial scar. It has now become apparent that even at rest, patients with severe coronary stenosis may show redistribution of thallium, which can be detected only by serial imaging (Fig. 7-12). Serial imaging may be helpful in identifying the site and extent of myocardial ischemia in patients with unstable angina, and in peri-infarction ischemia in patients with no

L   R

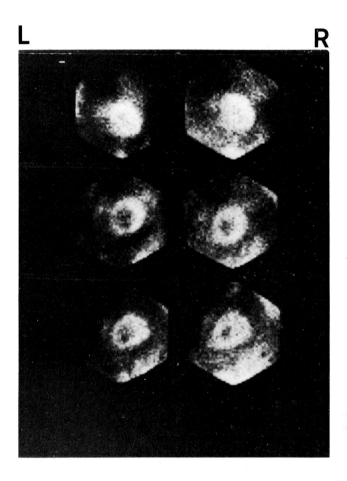

Figure 7-10.   Exercise thallium-201 study on a patient with 100 percent stenosis of the RCA and 80 percent stenosis of the LAD as seen on angiography. (Initial images, left; two-hour delayed redistribution images, right; anterior, 45° LAO, 60° LAO projections from top, middle bottom). The delayed images have been "count normalized" to the initial images. On the initial images there is increased pulmonary activity, a thin inferior wall (anterior view), a thin septum with defect (45° LAO), and a defect in the right ventricle (45° and 60° LAO). On the delayed images there is (1) partial redistribution into the inferior and septal walls, but (2) not into the right ventricle. These findings indicate (1) septal and inferior left ventricular ischemia, and (2) right ventrical scar.

myocardial infarction.[22-24] In patients with acute myocardial infarction, the extent to which thallium-201 redistribution occurs may be an indication of a zone of myocardium that may be in jeopardy but which could be protected by aggressive therapeutic intervention. The importance of this observation is that the presence of a myocardial defect on the images

L   R

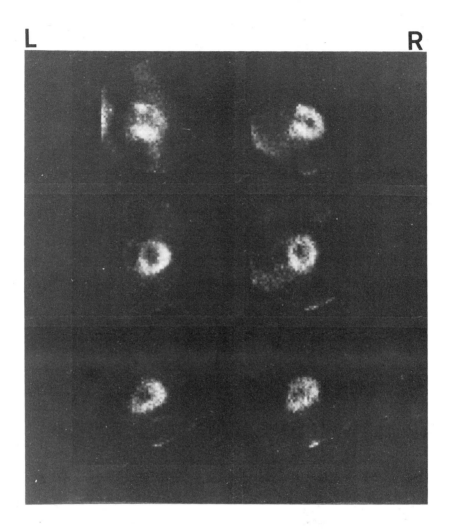

Figure 7-11. Exercise thallium-201 study on a patient with 99 percent stenosis of the proximal LAD, 100 percent stenosis of the LAD, 30 percent stenosis of the RCA, and 50 percent circumflex stenosis on coronary arteriography (initial images, left; two-hour delayed redistribution images, right; anterior, 45° LAO, 60° LAO projections, top, middle, bottom). In addition to the slightly increased pulmonary activity immediately after injection, there is a transient high septal defect seen on the 45° and 60° LAO projections characteristics of exercise induced ischemia. The exercise stress test was terminated because of anginal pain and ischemic ECG changes.

of a patient injected with thallium-201 while at rest is not necessarily indicative of scar. When decreased regional uptake of thallium-201 is noted on myocardial images, redistribution imaging is required regardless of whether the tracer was injected while the patient was resting or exercising.

L   R

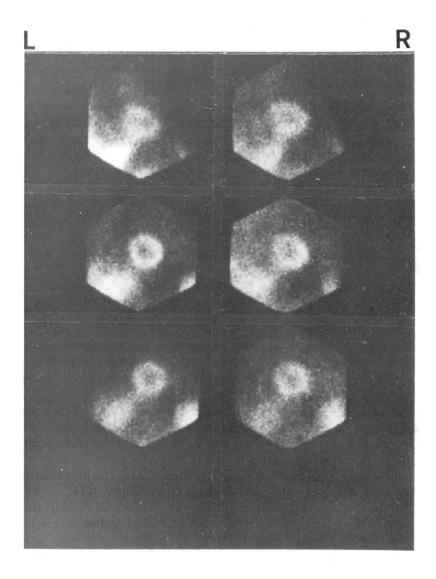

Figure 7-12. Thallium-201 study injected at rest in a patient with unstable angina pectoris; 90 percent stenosis of LAD and 40 percent stenosis of RCA were demonstrated on angiogrpahy (initial images, left; two-hour delayed redistribution images, right; anterior, 45° LAO, 60° LAO projections, top, middle, bottom). On the initial anterior image there is a low anterior lateral wall defect which is filled in two hours later on the delayed study. The observation of myocardial thallium-201 redistribution in patients at rest as well as exercising, indicates the need to take delayed images of any patient who exhibits myocardial perfusion abnormalities initially. The presence of a myocardial thallium-201 defect seen in the scan of a patient indicates either a scar or ischemia, and thus delayed imaging is required to differentiate one from the other.

References

1. Zaret, B.L., Strauss, H.W., Martin, N.D., et al.: Noninvasive regional myocardial perfusion with radioactive potassium. *N Engl J Med* **288**:809, 1973.

2. Holman, B.L.: Radionuclide methods in the evaluation of myocardial ischemia and infarction. *Circulation* **53**(Suppl I) :I, 1976.

3. Ritchie, J.L., Trobaugh, G.B., Hamilton, G.W., et al.: Myocardial imaging with thallium-201 at rest and during exercise: Comparison with coronary arteriography and resting and stress electrocardiography. *Circulation* **56**:67, 1977.

4. Trobaugh, G.B., Ritchie, J.L., and Hamilton, G.W.: Rest exercise imaging in coronary artery disease. In Ritchie, J.L., Hamilton, G.W., and Wackers, J. Th. (Eds.): *Thallium-201 Myocardial Imaging.* New York, Raven Press, 1978.

5. Berman, D.S., Salel, A.F., DeNardo, G.L., et al.: Noninvasive detection of regional myocardial ischemia using rubidium 81 and the scintillation camera: Comparison with stress electrocardiography in patients with arteriographically documented coronary stenosis. *Circulation* **52**:619,1975.

6. Sapirstein, L.A., et al.: Regional blood flow by fractional indicators. *Am J Physiol* **193**:161, 1958.

7. Gehring, P.J., and Hammond, P.B.: The interrelationship between thallium and potassium in animals. *J Pharmacol Exp Ther* **155**:187,1967.

8. Lebowitz, E., Green, M.W., Bradley-Moore, P., et al.: Thallium-201 for medical use, *J Nucl Med* **14**:421, 1973.

9. Britten, J.S., and Blank, M.: Thallium activation of the (Na^+-K^+) - activated ATPase of rabbit kidney. *Biochim Biophys Acta* **159**:160, 1968.

10. Welch, H.F., Strauss, H.W., and Pitt, B.: The extraction of thallium-201 by the myocardium. *Circulation* **56**:188, 1977.

11. Gould, K.L., Lopscomb, K., and Hamilton, G.W.: Physiologic basis for assessing critical coronary stenosis. *Am J Cardiol* **33**:87, 1974.

12. Pohost, G.M., Zir, L.M., Moore, R.H., et al.: Differentiation of transiently ischemic from infarcted myocardium by serial imaging after a single dose of thallium-201. *Circulation* **55**:294, 1977.

13. Osborn, R.C., and Smitherman, T.C.: Differentiation of transiently ischemic from infarcted myocardium following acute myocardial ischemia in man by serial myocardial scintigraphy following a single dose of thallium-201. *Clin Res* (abstract), 1977.

14. Hor, G., Sebenig, H., Sauer, E., et al.: Thallium-201 redistribution in coronary heart disease. *J Nucl Med* **18**:599, 1977.

15. Beller,G.A., and Pohost, G.M.: Mechanism for thallium-201 redistribution after transient myocardial ischemia. *Circulation* **55**, **56**(Suppl III):140, 1977.

16. Schelbert, H., Schuler, G., Ashburn, W., et al.: Time course of redistribution of thallium-201 after transient ischemia. *J Nucl Med* **18**:598, 1977.

17. Schwartz, J.S., Ponto, R., Carlyle, P., et al.: Early redistribution of thallium-201 after temporary ischemia. *Circulation* **57**:332, 1978.

18. Gewirtz, H., O'Keefe, D.D., Pohost, G.M., et al.: The effect of ischemia on thallium-201 clearance from the myocardium. *Circulation* **58**:215, 1978.

19. Botvinick, E.H., Taradash, M.R., Shames, D.M., et al.: Thallium-201 myocardial perfusion scintigraphy for the clinical clarification of normal, abnormal and equivocal electrocardiographic stress tests. *Am J Cardiol* **41**:43, 1978.

20. Bingham, J.B., Strauss, H.W., Pohost, G.M., et al.: Mechanisms of lung uptake of thallium-201. *Circulation* **57**, **58** (Suppl II), 1978.

21. Cook, D.J., Bailey, I., Strauss, H.W., et al.: Thallium-201 for myocardial imaging: Appearance of the normal heart. *J Nucl Med* **17**:583, 1976.

22. Maseri, A., L'Abbate, A., Pesola, A., et al.: Regional myocardial perfusion in patients with atherosclerotic coronary artery disease, at rest and during angina pectoris induced by tachycardia. *Circulation* **55**:423, 1977.

23. Wackers, F.J., Sokole, E.B., Samson, G., et al.: Value and limitations of thallium-201 scintigraphy in acute phase of myocardial infarction. *N Eng J Med* **295**:1, 1976.

24. Maseri, A., L'Abbate, A., Baroldi, G., et al.: Coronary vasospasm as a possible cause of myocardial infarction. *N Eng J Med* **299**:1271, 1979.

CHAPTER VIII

Myocardial Perfusion Imaging in Ischemic Heart Disease: A Clinician's Viewpoint

Michael H. Keelan, Jr., M.D.
Jagmeet S. Soin, M.D.
Harold L. Brooks, M.D.

Coronary artery disease is clearly a major health concern in this country. Acute myocardial infarction or sudden death are too often the first clinical expressions of the disease. Even after a coronary event has occurred it is frequently difficult to evaluate an individual patient's probability of further attacks. Initially, clinicians relied on the history of anginal chest pain or an abnormal electrocardiogram to identify the patient with coronary heart disease. History of classical angina pectoris alone accurately predicts the presence of obstructive coronary disease in 85 to 95 percent of cases.[1] This important observation is tempered by the recognition that nearly 50 percent of patients with coronary artery disease fail to develop significant angina prior to myocardial infarction or sudden death. The resting electrocardiogram has gross limitations and we now rely most frequently on the exercise electrocardiogram as the primary noninvasive test for (1) identifying latent coronary disease in asymptomatic patients, (2) evaluating patients with chest pain, (3) following patients after myocardial infarction, and (4) following patients after coronary bypass surgery. The widespread availability and use of coronary arteriography has allowed us to correlate anatomic studies with the noninvasive testing procedures. The sensitivity (number of true positive/number of true positive + the number of false negative) reflects the ability of the test to identify accurately the patient who has the disease in question. Specificity (number of true negative/number of true negative + number of false positive) is an index of the test's ability to predict accurately the absence of the disease. The ideal screening test for coronary disease should minimize the numbers of both false positive and false negative studies.

Correlation of graded exercise electrocardiogram tests with coronary angiographic studies has shown repeatedly that sensitivity is a function of the number of major vessels with significant stenosis.[2] Thus, only about 50 percent of the patients with significant stenosis of a single vessel (greater than 70 percent lumen occlusion) demonstrate ST segment depression with exercise, while 80 to 90 percent of patients with significant stenosis of three vessels display diagnostic changes of ischemia. Moreover, specificity of the changes in the ST segment with effort depends upon the population being tested. In patients with typical angina pectoris, depression of the ST segment correctly identifies coronary heart disease 90 to 95 percent of the time. Conversely, false positive ST segment depression is a well recognized clinical problem. A significant percentage of young and middle-aged females with atypical chest pain syndromes may show such changes. False positive tests constitute a major shortcoming of the exercise electrocardiogram. Misdiagnosis of coronary artery disease in this setting may lead to a lifelong cardiac neurosis. It is apparent, therefore that the diagnostic value of the stress electrocardiogram has distinct limitations, a topic recently addressed by Epstein and Redwood.[3]

The combination of graded exercise testing with radionuclide injection was introduced by Zaret et al. using ^{43}K as a myocardial imaging agent.[4] Potassium-43 and other monovalent cations distribute in myocardium in proportion to the regional myocardial perfusion. Thallium-201 (^{201}Tl), currently the most widely used agent, is produced in a cyclotron by irradiating natural thallium targets with 31 meV protons. The nuclear reaction is ^{201}Tl (p, 3n) Pb which has a 9.4 hour half-life. The lead-201 (^{201}Pb) is the parent of ^{201}Tl. Thallium-201 decays by electron capture with a 73-hour half-life. It emits mercury K characteristic x-rays of 69 to 83 keV in 98 percent abundance and gamma rays of 135 to 167 keV in 10 percent of total abundance. The lower energy peak is used for clinical imaging. Thallium-201 is distributed to the myocardium in proportion to the amount of blood flowing to the myocardium and its extraction by the myocardial cell depends upon active transport across the myocardial cell membrane requiring membrane adenosine triphosphatase (ATPase).[5] In most instances, the myocardial extraction depends on regional perfusion, although theoretically a decrease in uptake of the radiotracer might reflect a regional defect of membrane transport, independent of blood flow.

The focal nature of coronary atherosclerosis results in regional myocardial perfusion deficits. The extent of the perfusion defect is related to the severity of the arterial stenosis, the portion of the perfusion bed affected and its viability, and the degree of coronary collateral flow. Localized perfusion defects are readily identified as "cold" spots on a thallium perfusion scan. Defects on a resting scan reflect decreased myocardial uptake due to fibrosis or severe ischemia. Areas of potential ischemia are identified when myocardial blood flow demands are accentuated, as they are during exercise. Consistent resolution of such defects by radionuclide techniques would clearly represent a major advance in the noninvasive diagnosis of significant obstructive coronary artery disease.

Technique

Optimal nuclear imaging of any organ depends upon a high target-to-background count ratio. Stressing the patient to maximum effort or as close as possible to predicted maximum heart rate in the fasting state assures slightly higher myocardial blood flow and decreased hepatic blood flow. The importance of reaching an adequate exercise level cannot be overly emphasized. McLaughlin et al.[6] demonstrated that the reproducibility of results was strikingly reduced when the level of exercise was reduced.

A systemic vein is cannulated before the patient begins to exercise and a bolus of 1.5 to 2.0 millicuries of thallium-201 is injected during the final minute of exercise. The blood pressure, pulse, and electrocardiogram are continuously monitored during the exercise. The defibrillator and other resuscitative equipment are always kept at hand. Cardiac medications may be withheld so that electrocardiogram changes accompanying the stress perfusion scan may be assessed; however, studies made by Welsh, Strauss, and Pitt have demonstrated no significant adverse effect on perfusion studies of patients who had taken digitalis or propranolol.[5] Experimental work by Costin and Zaret[7] has raised some question regarding the effect of propranolol, however, and that medication probably should be discontinued whenever possible at least 48 hours before the study.

Thallium-201 is taken up and redistributed quickly in the myocardium. Most myocardial uptake is noted in the first two to five minutes. The maximum myocardial-to-background ratio is achieved at 10 to 15 minutes after injection and this ratio stays constant for two hours. The thallium clears the myocardial tissue slowly, with 50 percent activity remaining in the myocardium after 24 hours, and 15 percent remaining at the end of the fifth day. The slow clearance puts a practical limitation on repeat study, which should be done at least one week after the initial study. Imaging should be started as soon as possible after the radio-nuclide has been injected and exercise has been terminated. Five min-utes is an optimal interval and any further delay before scanning may reduce the diagnostic yield because of redistribution of the radioisotope.

The myocardial images are done in at least three projections: anterior, 45° left anterior oblique and 60° left anterior oblique. Generally, an Anger scintillation camera is used because of its good spatial resolution. Any standard field of view camera with 37 photomultiplier tubes is satisfactory. The multicrystal imaging device can also be used. Another important factor is the choice of collimator. A combination of increased spatial resolution and reasonable sensitivity is required to measure small amounts of radioactivity present in the myocardium. We recommend the images taken with a low energy all-purpose (LEAP) or a high resolution collimator. However, if the "R" wave portion of the electrocardiogram is synchronized with the images of the thallium study, the use of a high sensitivity collimator is mandatory.[8]

Perfusion scans are interpreted using direct visual inspection with or without computer enhancement of the images. Figure 8-1 shows a typical normal unprocessed thallium myocardial perfusion study obtain-ed following exercise. Perfusion zones are divided according to the anatomic distribution of the major coronary arteries. This technique is described in Chapter 5. Perfusion defects that can be detected only after exercise indicate ischemia. If the defect can still be detected in a resting state, it probably is a myocardial scar or infarction. The delayed study may be done three to four hours after the initial post exercise images, thereby eliminating the need for another patient visit as well as a subsequent injection of thallium. Thallium myocardial redistribution is considered in detail in Chapter 7. An alternate technique requires the patient to return on another day for a resting study. The stress perfusion scan is generally done first, since a negative study would eliminate the need for a resting scan.

Clinical Value of Myocardial Perfusion Imaging

What, then, is the role of perfusion scintigraphy in the assessment of patients with suspected coronary artery disease? How does it comple-ment history and stress electrocardiography in the overall evaluation process? Combined stress electrocardiography and cardiac perfusion scintigraphy have been correlated with coronary arteriography to eval-uate patients with known or suspected coronary heart disease.

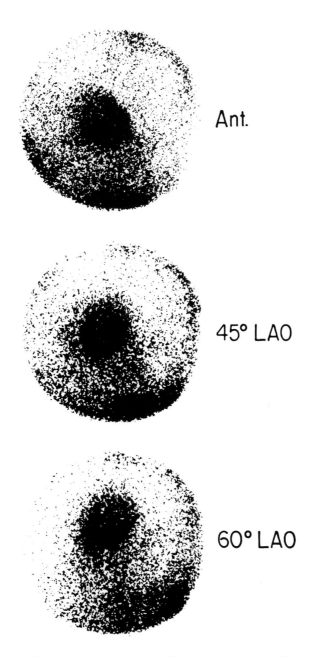

Figure 8-1.   Normal exercise thallium-201 perfusion scan. Uniform distribution to all segments of the myocardium.

In patients with chest pain (angina or nonangina), but no prior myocardial infarction, Turner et al. found the overall sensitivity of the stress perfusion scan to be no different from that of the stress electrocardiogram (68 percent versus 71 percent). A history of classical angina pectoris more accurately predicted the presence of significant obstructive coronary disease than either noninvasive test. Data were not analyzed to determine the number of vessels diseased.[9] A number of other individuals and multicenter studies have reported greater overall sensitivity of stress perfusion scintigraphy.[10-12] However, a high percentage of the patients described in the latter studies had abnormalities apparent on resting electrocardiograms, a condition known to diminish the sensitivity of the exercise electrocardiogram. Bailey et al. found 62 percent of patients with abnormal resting electrocardiograms had new perfusion defects and only 38 percent had new ST segment changes.[10] They also demonstrated improved sensitivity in detecting single vessel obstructive coronary disease. A typical case of single vessel disease is illustrated in Figure 8-2. This 55 year old patient had atypical chest pain and a negative stress electrocardiogram. An abnormal ^{201}Tl scan prompted study of the coronary arteries. This study revealed stenosis of the right coronary artery. Similarly, Botvinick et al.[12] emphasized the value of the stress scintigram in evaluating patients with abnormal or equivocal electrocardiograms.

The stress perfusions scan aids in detecting new ischemic disease in patients with previous myocardial damage as evidenced by abnormal resting scans or abnormal resting electrocardiograms. Figure 8-3 illustrates the presence of new perfusion defects in a patient with old anterior myocardial infarction. Ritchie et al. warn that stress perfusion scans do not adequately predict individual stenotic arteries in patients with multiple vessel disease.[11] In other words, detection of a single perfusion defect is not uncommon even in patients with the presence of angiographically proven obstructive disease in several vessels. The case illustrated in Figure 8-4 clarifies this point. The patient had decreased perfusion only in the septal region; whereas severe obstructive disease was noted in the left anterior descending and left circumflex arteries. This fact is noteworthy if the stress scintigram is to be used to follow patients who have had myocardial infarctions. Present data are inadequate to conclude that the stress scintigram is a sufficiently sensitive test to exclude multivessel disease in patients with a previous myocardial infarction.

Finally, several recent reports have described the role of preoperative and postoperative stress scintigraphy for evaluating graft patency. Thallium-201 myocardial perfusion provides a reasonable and objective noninvasive technique for evaluating the patency of aortocoronary bypass

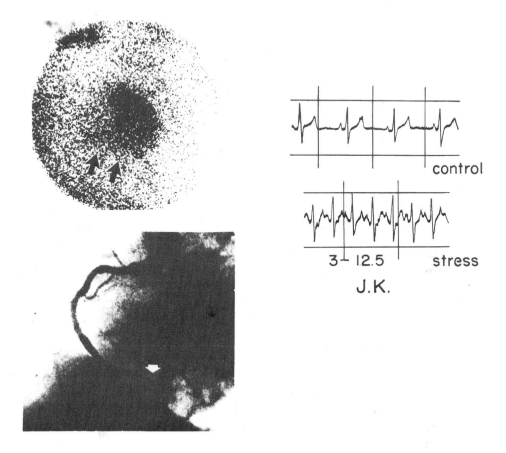

control

3 ⊥ 12.5   stress

J.K.

Figure 8-2. Abnormal perfusion of inferior wall in 50 year old male with recurrent chest pain, negative stress ECG. Right coronary angiogram demonstrated distal RCA high grade stenosis.

graft. Before surgery it is desirable to have myocardial perfusion scans taken after exercise, so that they are available for comparison with postoperative scans. Various investigators have reported that areas of normal thallium perfusion correlate well with patent graft to that region. Conversely, all patients demonstrating defects have associated graft dysfunction.[13]

Perfusion defects may not be detected in patients with significant coronary lesions for any of several reasons. Inadequate exercise has already been implicated. Another source of insensitivity is uniform or global ventricular ischemia. This occurs most commonly in patients with left main coronary artery stenosis. Fortunately, the electrocardiogram is sensitive to the presence of such disease. The severity of symptoms may

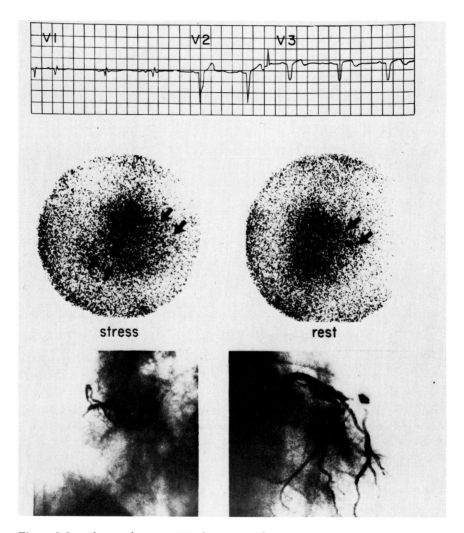

Figure 8-3. Abnormal resting ECG (anterior MI), extensive anterior and inferior exercise perfusion defects with incomplete late reperfusion. Total occlusion of RCA with severe stenosis of LAD branch of LCA and collateral to RCA.

also dictate the need for further evaluation. In the patients with multivessel disease, new perfusion defects are often demonstrated, but because there are differences in perfusion in a number of areas, not all zones of decreased perfusion can be accurately identified by visual inspection. How sensitive the study is depends on where the area of ischemia is located.

Most reported studies cite a specificity which is superior to that

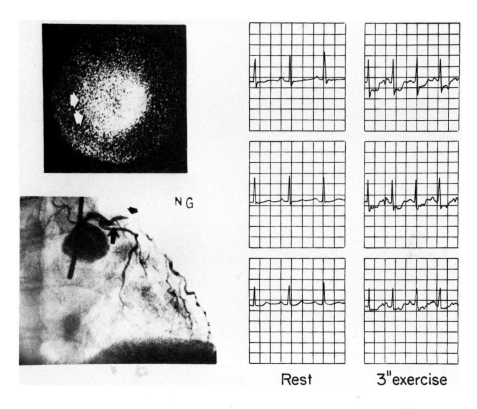

Figure 8-4. Decreased septal perfusion but normal inferior and posterior perfusion in patient with total occlusion of LAD and severe stenosis in large circumflex branch of LCA.

described for the stress electrocardiogram. Stress electrocardiograms are influenced by metabolic, electrolyte, and drug effects. Changes so induced account for a significant number of false positive interpretations. This clinical problem occurs most commonly when the stress electrocardiogram is done as a screening procedure for patients who are asymptomatic or have atypical, nonischemic pain. The specificity of the myocardial perfusion scan is sufficiently high (85 to 90 percent) to allow recognition of the electrocardiographic inaccuracy in most instances. False positive stress thallium scans have been reported in association with cardiomyopathy and mitral valve prolapse syndrome.[14]

Indications for ^{201}Tl Myocardial Perfusion Study

Based on the currently available data, thallium myocardial perfusion imaging appears most useful in evaluating: (1) patients with atypical chest pain syndromes, particularly when pain is believed to be nonischemic—many patients in this category will have false positive stress electrocardiograms and are identified correctly by a normal stress perfusion study; (2) patients suspected of having additional coronary artery disease, who have abnormal resting electrocardiograms. It is well known that the stress electrocardiogram is not as reliable for patients with grossly abnormal electrocardiograms. Pre-existing intraventricular conduction defects, old myocardial infarction, or resting ST-T changes may make it impossible to recognize ischemic changes during exertion. Exercise perfusion scanning eliminates the need to rely on electrocardiographic criteria alone. Patients with "suspicious" or equivocal changes in ST segment of electrocardiograms may be better evaluated with exercise scintigrams. However, additional obstructive disease may not be well recognized in all instances and consequently the failure to demonstrate more than a single perfusion defect in a patient who has had a myocardial infarction does not necessarily exclude multiple vessel disease; (3) patients who are studied preoperatively and postoperatively to evaluate graft patency.

In patients with classical angina pectoris, but who have not had myocardial infarctions, the scintigram has greater sensitivity than the stress electrocardiogram, particularly if the disease is limited to one vessel. Since history alone is more sensitive than either the stress electrocardiogram or the stress scintigram, negative studies do not preclude the diagnosis of ischemic coronary artery disease. At present, stress perfusion scintigraphy is not recommended for the "screening" of asymptomatic patients. Routine studies should be limited to those asymptomatic patients with positive stress electrocardiograms. A summary of our approach to a patient with chest pain is presented in Figure 8-5.

Conclusions

1. Stress electrocardiography has significant limitations of sensitivity and specificity. Single vessel coronary artery disease and abnormalities on resting electrocardiograms are major factors affecting the sensitivity of the electrocardiogram. Metabolic, pharmacologic, and electrolyte changes influence the ST-T segments and may result in false positive electrocardiograms, thereby reducing the specificity.

2. Exercise thallium-201 studies offer better sensitivity and specificity in the diagnosis of coronary artery disease. Increased sensitivity is most significant in patients with single vessel disease or abnormalities on

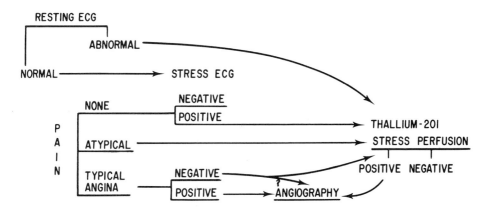

Figure 8-5. A proposed scheme for evaluating patients with chest pain.

resting electrocardiograms. The high degree of specificity elminates the need for invasive studies in many patients with "false positive" stress electrocardiograms.

3. Factors that can compromise the results of this technique are inadequate exercise, global ischemia, large resting perfusion abnormalities, or small perfusion deficits.

4. The role of thallium perfusion scans has not yet been clearly defined in the evaluation of patients with classical angina.

5. Cost limitations at the present time dictate that thallium-201 studies be done only to obtain specific information not clearly available from the standard stress electrocardiogram.

References

1. Friesinger, G.C., and Smith, R.F.: Correlation of electrocardiographic studies and arteriographic findings with angina pectoris. *Circulation* **46**:1173-1184, 1973.

2. Farris, J.V., McHenry, P.L., and Morris, S.N.: Concepts and applications of treadmill exercise testing and the exercise electrocardiogram. *Am Heart J* **95**:102, 1978.

3. Redwood, D. R., Borer, J.S., and Epstein, S.E.: Whither the ST segment during exercise. *Circulation* **54**:703-706, 1976.

4. Zaret, B.L., Strauss, H. W., Martin, N.D., et al.: Noninvasive regional myocardial perfusion with radioactive potassium: Study of patients at rest, exercise and during angina pectoris. *N Engl J Med* **288**:809-813, 1973.

5. Weich, H.F., Strauss, H.W., and Pitt, B.: The extraction of thallium-201 by

the myocardium. *Circulation* **56**:188-191, 1977.

6. McLaughlin, P.R., Martin, R.P., Doherty, P., et al.: Reproducibility of thallium-201 myocardial imaging. *Circulation* **55**:497-503, 1977.

7. Costin, J.D., and Zaret, B. L.: Effect of propranolol and digitalis upon radioactive thallium and potassium uptake in myocardial and skeletal muscle. *J Nucl Med* **17**:535, 1976 (Abstract).

8. Coleman, A., Hamilton, G.W., and Robertson, M.: Thallium-201 myocardial imaging—technique and equipment for clinical rest-exercise imaging. *Applied Radiology/ Nuclear Medicine*, Jan-Feb:165-168, 1978.

9. Turner, D.A., Battle, W.E., Deshmukh, H., et al.: The predictive value of myocardial perfusion scintigraphy after stress in patients without previous myocardial infarction. *J Nucl Med* **19**:249-255, 1978.

10. Bailey, I.K., Griffith, L.S., Rouleau, J.R., et al.: Thallium-201 myocardial perfusion imaging at rest and during exercise: Comparative sensitivity to electrocardiography in coronary artery disease. *Circulation* **55**:79-87, 1977.

11. Ritchie, J.L., Trobaugh, G.B., Hamilton, G.W., et al.: Myocardial imaging with thallium-201 at rest and during exercise: Comparison with coronary arteriography and resting and stress electrocardiography. *Circulation* **56**:66-71, 1977.

12. Botvinick, E.H., Taradash, M.R., Shames, D.M., et al.: Thallium-201 myocardial perfusion scintigraphy for the clinical clarification of normal, abnormal, and equivocal electrocardiographic stress tests. *Am J Cardiol* **41**:43-48, 1978.

13. Ritchie, J.L., Narahara, K.A., Trobaugh, G.B., et al.: Thallium-201 myocardial imaging before and after coronary revascularization. Assessment of regional myocardial blood flow and graft patency. *Circulation* **56**:830-836, 1977.

14. Tresch, D.D., Soin, J.S., Siegel, R., et al.: Mitral valve prolapse, evidence for a myocardial perfusion abnormality. *Am J Cardiol* **41**:441, 1978 (Abstract).

CHAPTER IX

Myocardial Perfusion Imaging in Nonatherosclerotic Cardiac Disorders

Donald D. Tresch, M.D.
Jagmeet S. Soin, M.D.
Harold L. Brooks, M.D.

Thallium-201 scintigraphy is used primarily in the detection and evaluation of coronary artery disease. However, it can be useful in evaluating other cardiac disease processes. Perfusion defects caused by other cardiac diseases will show up on thallium-201 scans as areas of decreased uptake in the myocardium. Disease processes causing myocardial hypertrophy will show up on thallium-201 scans as areas of increased uptake.

Myocardial Infiltrative Processes

The distribution of thallium-201 in the heart reflects myocardial perfusion, and thallium-201 scintigraphy has proved sensitive in detecting abnormal coronary blood flow. But a perfusion defect does not always indicate ischemic disease. Destruction or damage to myocardial cells by an infiltrative process, such as tumor, granuloma or amyloidosis, may result in a perfusion defect. In such instances, the decreased uptake of thallium may represent alterations in cation transport in the myocardium, independent of regional blood flow.

Recent studies have demonstrated that thallium-201 imaging of the myocardium can be useful in evaluating myocardium in patients with pulmonary sarcoidosis.[1] Pulmonary hypertension may cause hypertrophy and dilation of the right ventricle in these patients. With granulomatosis displacement of myocardial cells, scattered perfusion defects will be seen

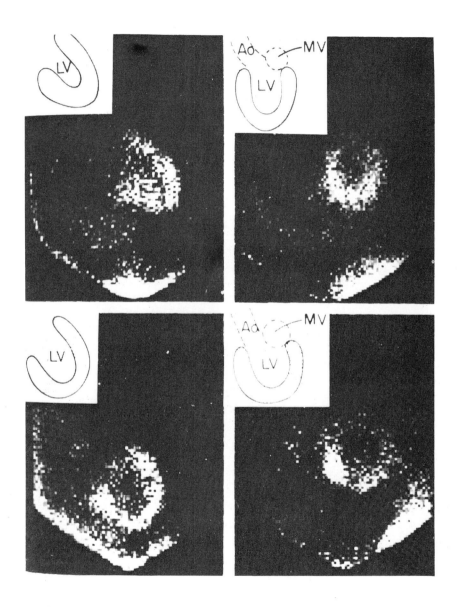

Figure 9-1. Thallium-201 myocardial perfusion images in normal (top), and in a patient with cardiac sarcoidosis (bottom). The abnormal decreased perfusion is noted in the posterior wall on the LAO 45° view. (Reproduced with permission from Bulkley, B.H., et al.: The use of thallium-201 for myocardial perfusion imaging in sarcoid heart disease. *Chest* **72**: 27-32, 1977).

on thallium-201 myocardial imaging (Fig. 9-1). Clinical autopsy studies have shown such myocardial infiltration may occur in patients with no clinical evidence of sarcoidosis. Since myocardial sarcoid can be treated with steroids, detection by thallium-201 scintigraphy may be valuable in instituting therapy early.

Left Ventricular Hypertrophy

Cardiac enlargement can be readily demonstrated by thallium-201 imaging. Not only can dimensions be evaluated, but often the findings suggest certain pathologic disorders. Left ventricular volume and pressure overload disorders may be distinguished by the relative mass of muscle in comparison to the size of the chamber. Primary pressure overload increases the thickness of the heart wall while chamber size remains normal. Thus on thallium imaging, the mural image appears more intense in comparison to the chamber image. In contrast, left ventricular volume overload causes an increase in chamber size with a proportionate increase in thickness of the left ventricular wall. Therefore, imaging in such cases usually reveals a normal distribution of thallium, although over a larger area. As the disease progresses, left ventricular ejection fraction is reduced and the cavity becomes more prominent in comparison to the left ventricular wall.

In certain cases of congestive heart failure with cardiac enlargement, thallium-201 scintigraphy may be useful in differentiating ischemia and nonischemic cardiomyopathies. In a patient with an ischemic cardiomyopathy due to diffuse coronary artery disease, thallium-201 scintigraphy reveals a dilated left ventricular cavity with absent or spotty myocardial thallium uptake; whereas, in a patient with a primary nonischemic cardiomyopathy, thallium-201 imaging will demonstrate relatively uniform thallium-201 uptake without, or with only small focal defects involving less than 20 percent of the ventricular circumference. Although this finding of a spotty uptake of thallium-201 is characteristic of an ischemic cardiomyopathy, such defects can also be seen in an infiltrative process in the myocardium. However, the size of focal perfusion defects are usually much greater in an ischemic cardiomyopathy, usually over 20 percent of the circumference of the left ventricle.[2]

Right Ventricular Hypertrophy

Clinically, right ventricular hypertrophy is not always easy to detect, although its detection can be important in the diagnosis and management of a critically ill patient. Electrocardiographic, radiographic and echocardiographic findings are not always reliable in making the diagnosis of right ventricular hypertrophy. Recently, Cohen[3] has reported that right ventricular hypertrophy can be detected with thallium-201 scintigraphy more reliably than with routine electrocardiography, especially in patients having combined right and left ventricular hypertrophy.

In normal individuals thallium-201 activity is absent in the right ventricle or barely visible due to the thinner right ventricular wall as compared to the larger left ventricular wall. It may also reflect the lower myocardial blood flow per gram of muscle in the right ventricular wall. This low level of thallium activity in the right ventricle cannot be distinguished from background activity on equipment presently available. However, in the presence of right ventricular hypertrophy, thallium activity is seen in the right ventricular wall on the resting scintigram and, with long-standing pulmonary hypertension, a right ventricle of greater than 1 cm of thickness can usually be seen in the left anterior oblique image (Fig. 9-2). The relative thickness of both the right and left ventricular myocardium can also be determined by thallium scanning.[4] Increased uptake of thallium by a hypertrophied right ventricle is nonspecific and gives no information regarding the cause of the hypertrophy.

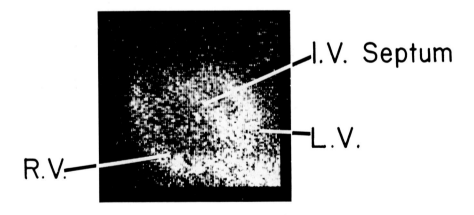

Figure 9-2.   An anterior thallium myocardial perfusion image obtained at rest in a patient with severe idiopathic pulmonary hypertension. Note the intense thallium activity in the dilated right ventricle.

Asymmetrical Septal Hypertrophy

Hypertrophy of the ventricular wall is not diagnostic for a specific disease. It may be secondary to hypertension or aortic valvular stenosis, or it may be a primary disorder due to a cardiomyopathy. In the former instance, left ventricular hypertrophy is concentric with uniform thickness of the free wall and septum of the left ventricle. The ratio of the thickness of the left ventricular wall to septum does not change even though hypertrophy occurs. In contrast, certain forms of primary cardiomyopathies produce asymmetric hypertrophy so that thickening of the apex and septum is disproportionate in comparison to the free wall of the left ventricle. Asymmetrical septal hypertrophy (ASH) has now been established as a distinguishing feature of the hypertrophic cardiomyopathies, including idiopathic hypertrophic subaortic stenosis (IHSS). Although ASH and IHSS is best diagnosed by echocardiography, occasionally such studies are not technically possible. Thallium-201 scintigraphy can be useful in such cases,[5] since thallium-201 imaging in the left anterior oblique projection will reveal a septum that is disproportionately thick when compared to the free wall of the left ventricle (Fig. 9-3). The ventricular cavity usually appears diminished in size.

Mitral Valve Prolapse

Patients with mitral valve prolapse are frequently bothered by chest pain and on occasion the pain may be similar to the angina pectoris of coronary atherosclerosis. The usefulness of thallium-201 to detect coronary artery disease in these individuals has been investigated with varying results. Massie[6] and Gaffney[7] have reported abnormal thallium imaging to be specific in distinguishing coronary atherosclerosis from mitral valve prolapse syndrome. In contrast, data from our laboratory[8] and from Staniloff[9] indicate that some patients with mitral valve prolapse syndrome and normal coronary arteriograms demonstrate significant perfusion defects. In our studies, patients with abnormal scans and normal coronary arteries showed more prominent associated clinical findings. It was not uncommon for these patients to have been hospitalized for severe chest pain simulating myocardial infarction. They frequently had abnormal exercise electrocardiograms and stress tests. The scintigrams in Figure 9-4 illustrate a case of mitral valve prolapse with abnormal myocardial perfusion and normal coronary arteriogram. We have postulated that in the absence of coronary artery disease, these perfusion abnormalities are caused by relative ischemia produced by the

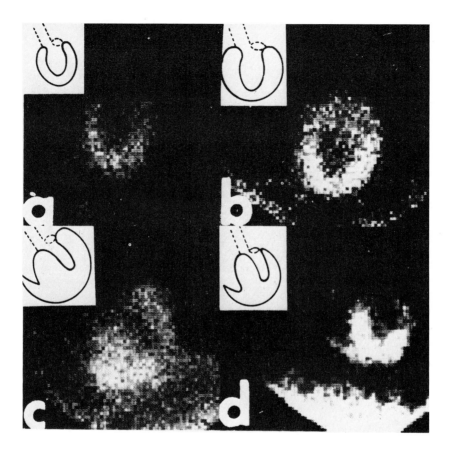

Figure 9-3. Thallium-201 myocardial perfusion studies in LAO 45° projection show (a) normal subject, (b) concentric hypertrophy of the left ventricle in a patient with hypertension, (c) obstructive cardiomyopathy, (d) nonobstructive cardiomyopathy. (Reproduced with permission from Bulkley, B.H., et al.: Idiopathic hypertrophic subaortic stenosis: Detection by thallium-201 myocardial perfusion imaging. *N Eng J Med* **293**: 1113-1116, 1975.)

undue traction applied to the myocardium by the prolapsing mitral valve apparatus.

Summary

While thallium-201 scintigraphy is used primarily in evaluating patients with coronary atherosclerosis, it is also useful in the assessment of certain nonatherosclerotic cardiac disease processes.

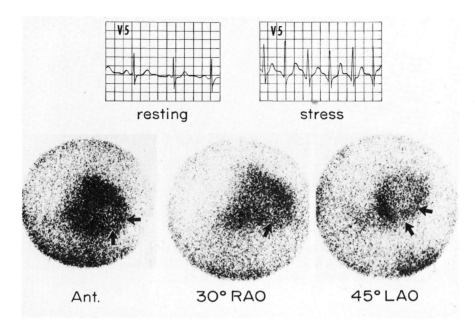

Figure 9-4. Thallium-201 myocardial perfusion study after exercise in a patient with mitral valve prolapse with normal coronary arteries. Note the decreased radioactivity in the posterior and inferior wall of the left ventricle.

These include:

      1. Myocardial Infiltrative Processes
      2. Left Ventricular Hypertrophy and Dilatation
      3. Right Ventricular Hypertrophy
      4. Certain Hypertrophic Cardiomyopathies
      5. Mitral Valve Prolapse Syndrome
      6. Ischemic and Nonischemic Cardiomyopathies

The exact role that thallium-201 scintigraphy can play in the clinical management of this patient population is currently under evaluation.

References

1. Bulkley, B.H., Rouleau, J.R., Whitaker, J.Q., et al.: The use of 201-thallium for myocardial perfusion imaging in sarcoid heart disease. *Chest* **72**:27-32, 1977.

2. Bulkley, B.H., Hutchins, G.M., Bailey, I., et al.: Thallium-201 imaging and gated cardiac pool scans in patients with ischemic and idiopathic cardiomyopathy: A clinical and pathologic study. *Circulation* **55**:753-760, 1977.

3. Cohen, H.A., Baird, M.G., Rouleau, J.R., et al.: Thallium-201 myocardial

imaging in patients with pulmonary hypertension. *Circulation* **54**:790-796, 1976.

4. Stevens, R.M., Baird, M.G., Fuhrmann, C.F., et al.: Detection of right ventricular hypertrophy by thallium-201 myocardial perfusion imaging. *Circulation* (Suppl II) **52**:243, 1975.

5. Bulkley, B.H., Rouleau, J.R, Strauss, H.W., et al.: Idiopathic hypertrophic subaortic stenosis: Detection by thallium-201 myocardial perfusion imaging. *N Engl J Med* **293**:1113-1116, 1975.

6. Massie, B., Botvinick, E., Shames, E., et al.: Myocardial perfusion scintigraphy in patients with mitral valve prolapse. *Circulation* **57**:19-26, 1978.

7. Gaffney, F.A., Wohl, A.W., Blomquist, C.G., et al.: Thallium-201 myocardial perfusion studies in patients with mitral valve prolapse syndrome. *Am J Med* **64**:21-26, 1978.

8. Tresch, D.D., Soin, J.S., Siegel, R., et al.: Mitral valve prolapse—Evidence for a myocardial perfusion abnormality. *Am J Cardiol* **41**:441, 1978.

9. Staniloff, H.M., Huckell, V.F., Morch, J.E., et al.: Abnormal myocardial perfusion defects in patients with mitral valve prolapse and normal coronary arteries. *Am J Cardiol* **41**:433, 1978.

CHAPTER X

Acute Myocardial Infarct Imaging Using Technetium-99m Pyrophosphate

*Robert W. Parkey, M.D., Fredrick J. Bonte, M.D.,
Samuel E. Lewis, M.D., L. Maximillian Buja, M.D.,
and James T. Willerson, M.D.*

There is a need for improved accuracy in diagnosing myocardial infarction. It is sometimes difficult to confirm the presence or absence of acute myocardial infarction in patients, despite the advances made in laboratory diagnosis of this entity. One or more of the following factors may make diagnosis difficult: (a) presence of an intraventricular conduction defect, such as left bundle branch block, (b) arrhythmias, (c) possible subendocardial necrosis, (d) delay in the patient's hospital admission after the onset of symptoms, or (e) previous infarcts in the same general location as the new damage. It is also difficult to distinguish between subendocardial ischemia and an acute subendocardial infarction using electrocardiographic findings alone. The recognition of acute myocardial infarcts in perioperative and postoperative periods following coronary artery revascularization is often difficult with traditional techniques.

With these considerations in mind, several groups throughout the country have worked over the past few years to develop noninvasive radionuclide imaging techniques that allow the physician to identify an acute myocardial infarct and to document its impact on ventricular performance.

This chapter deals with the technique that demonstrates acute myocardial necrosis. The role of myocardial perfusion dependent agents, such as thallium-201, in the detection of acute myocardial infarction and ventricular function studies will be discussed elsewhere.

Technetium-99m Phosphate Imaging

Although many agents have shown some affinity for acute necrotic myocardium,[2,11,13,14] technetium-99m stannous pyrophosphate (^{99m}Tc PYP) has so far been the most useful agent clinically.[2-7,9,12,17-28,34,39] We have been using this agent in a clinical setting for the last four years, and believe the ^{99m}Tc PYP scintigrams are a sensitive indicator of acute myocardial necrosis; however, several important factors must be kept in mind in order to obtain satisfactory clinical results:

1. The pathophysiology of an acute myocardial infarction is constantly changing and the results of any imaging test depend on the time and stage of infarction.
2. Since there is a changing pathophysiology, serial imaging should be done.
3. Quality control of the radiopharmaceuticals must be closely monitored because any labeling of the blood pool quickly destroys the accuracy of the test.

History and Mechanisms of Localization

Shen, Jennings, and D'Agostino[8,33] observed that calcium is deposited in subcrystalline and crystalline forms in irreversibly damaged myocardial cells. Their discovery led Bonte and associates[2] to suggest that because of the way pyrophosphate combines with crystalline or subcrystalline forms of calcium, technetium-99m pyrophosphate might be used in imaging to identify irreversibly damaged cells. Figure 10-1 demonstrates the animal originally studied. Figure 10-1A represents the control; B, the injection of mercury into the left anterior descending coronary artery, causing a large infarction in the anterior wall; C, after the injection of ^{99m}Tc PYP, the region of infarction was easily seen on routine scintigrams taken one to six days later; and D, increased concentration of ^{99m}Tc PYP in damaged myocardium disappeared within eight days after the myocardial infarct. This observation has led to extensive work with both human and animal models to define the exact mechanism and timing necessary for proper imaging, as well as to determine the efficacy of this imaging technique for identifying acute myocardial infarcts.

We have found that the three most important factors in determining ^{99m}Tc PYP uptake in the myocardium are:

1. The presence of irreversible cellular damage
2. Some residual blood flow back into the area of irreversible cellular damage

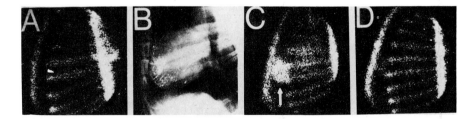

Figure 10-1. *A,* Lateral scintiphoto of the chest of a 20 kg dog made one hour after intravenous administration of 3.0 mCi Tc-99m stannous pyrophosphate (PYP). Only normal skeletal distribution is seen. *B,* Left lateral chest roentgenogram of animal seen in *A,* made immediately after the instillation of 0.1 ml metallic Hg into branches of the anterior descending artery. *C,* Left lateral scintiphoto of dog in *A* and *B* made 24 hours after Hg embolization (Fig. 10-1*B*) and one hour after intravenous administration of 3.0 mCi Tc-99m PYP. Note intense localization of radioactivity at a site (arrow) presumably coextant with a myocardial infarct (compare with Fig. 1-1*A*). *D,* Left lateral scintiphoto of same animal as seen in *A* and *C* made one hour after tracer administation, and eight days after infarction. Note that tracer localization has almost completely disappeared. Serial scintiphotos had shown persistent localization only through the fourth postinfarct day. (Reproduced from *Radiology* **110**:473-474, 1974. Used with permission of Radiological Society of North America.)

3. The length of time since infarct occurred and imaging was started

This last factor is dependent upon collateral blood flow. It has been shown that at least 3 grams of myocardial necrosis must exist before acute myocardial infarction can be identified consistently on scintigrams of animals with permanent coronary occlusion. In both animals and patients who have rapid flow back into the region of damaged tissues, there is an increased uptake of the phosphate. Such patients may have a temporary coronary occlusion, or possible infarction due to hypotension. Of these factors, the collateral flow into the injured tissue is probably the most important in determining the pattern seen scintigraphically. The variation in blood flow back into the injured tissue accounts for the "doughnut pattern" seen in some patients with large anterior and antero-lateral myocardial infarctions[5,30] (Fig. 10-2 and 10-3).

The mechanisms for concentration of ^{99m}Tc PYP in irreversibly damaged myocardium as described by Buja et al.[4-7] are outlined in Figure 10-4. Myocardial cells are injured by ischemia or other causes and membrane damage is accompanied by residual blood flow. Concentrations of electrolytes, including calcium, plasma proteins, and other plasma constituents, then change within the cell. The ^{99m}Tc phosphates, when injected under these conditions, have a strong association with the

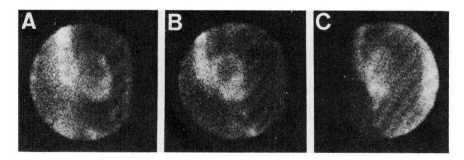

Figure 10-2.   Tc-99m PYP scintigrams in the anterior (*A*), left anterior oblique (*B*), and left lateral (*C*) projections in a patient with a large anterior wall myocardial infarction. Note the "doughnut" pattern caused from the pattern of collateral coronary blood flow at the time of imaging. (Reproduced from Willerson, J.T., et al.: *Circulation* **51**:1018, 1975. Used with permission of the American Heart Association, Inc.)

calcium deposits found in the injured cells; phosphate binding to macromolecules deposited in the injured myocardial cells may also be a factor.

Technique

There are several provisions for successful imaging of acute myocardial infarcts with ^{99m}Tc PYP. In laboratories where imaging with ^{99m}Tc PYP is done only occasionally, the quality control and timing are seldom perfect, and the test is usually of little value. Because the exact time of the patient's infarction is seldom known, a minimum of two examinations are needed to detect acute myocardial infarction with accuracy in the range of 95 percent. Imaging should be done as soon as possible after the patient is admitted to the cardiac unit, usually during the first day. If negative, serial scans should follow 48 hours apart; our experience has shown that the patient will have less than a 5 percent chance of another acute myocardial infarct. After considering the negative scans, serial electrocardiograms, and serial enzyme measurements, the clinician can be fairly confident that the patient does not have an acute myocardial infarction.

The main reason for serial imaging with this technique is the time required for collateral flow to enter the damaged tissue and allow for delivery of the radiopharmaceutical into the necrosed area. Figure 10-5 shows the value of serial imaging. The patient's image done on March 20 shows only a small blood pool. If this examination was the only one done

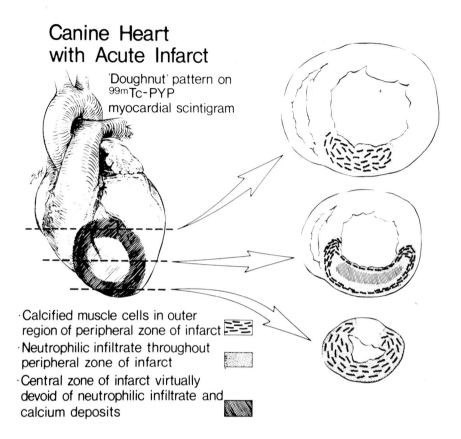

Canine Heart
with Acute Infarct

'Doughnut' pattern on
^{99m}Tc-PYP
myocardial scintigram

·Calcified muscle cells in outer
region of peripheral zone of infarct

·Neutrophilic infiltrate throughout
peripheral zone of infarct

·Central zone of infarct virtually
devoid of neutrophilic infiltrate and
calcium deposits

Figure 10-3.   Correlation of scintigrams and histologic features of a typical acute myocardial infarction produced in dogs by permanent occlusion of the proximal left anterior descending coronary artery. Histopathologic sections of transverse ventricular slices through the infarct reveal a large peripheral zone that is heavily infiltrated by neutophils that surround the subendocardially located central zone devoid of neutrophils. An area of extensive calcification of muscle cells is limited to the outer region of the peripheral zone of the infarct. The doughnut pattern observed on the Tc-99m PYP scintigram of the heart is explicable on the basis of selective concentation of Tc-99m PYP in this outer region of the peripheral zone of the infarct. (Reproduced from Buja, L.M., et al.: Morphologic correlates of technetium-99m stannous pyrophosphate imaging of acute myocardial infarcts in dogs. *Circulation* **52**: 596, 1975. Used with permission of the American Heart Association, Inc.)

on this patient, the scan would be called equivocal or negative. On additional images performed two days later, the blood flow entered the infarcted area and a large anterior wall doughnut-type lesion became apparent. Actually, earlier images were done on this patient on March 15, the day of his admission to the hospital. At this time, the patient had

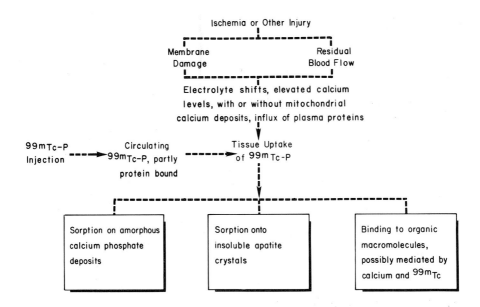

Figure 10-4. Proposed pathophysiologic basis for the scinitgraphic detection of tissue damage with Tc-99m PYP radiopharmaceuticals. (Reproduced with permission from Buja, L.M., et al.: *J Clin Invest* **60**:724-740, 1977.)

an infarct in the anterior apex of the myocardium. Chest pain recurred several days later and images were done on March 20. The large extension of infarct in the anterior wall of the myocardium became evident two days later. Note the resolution of the abnormal distribution of ^{99m}Tc PYP on April 19, approximately one month later. ^{99m}Tc PYP myocardial scans that are consistently positive will be discussed later in this chapter, but this example demonstrates how the phosphate scan can demonstrate a small lesion with later extension and be used to determine adequate collateral blood flow to the damaged area.

Most ^{99m}Tc PYP myocardial scintigrams are done two hours after the radionuclide injection. If unbound ^{99m}Tc pertechnetate (poor labeling) is injected with the ^{99m}Tc stannous pyrophosphate, the red cells will be quickly labelled and acute myocardial infarct imaging cannot be reliably done for at least 24 to 48 hours. For this reason, quality control is particularly important. Figure 10-6 shows how anterior and lateral views can help distinguish an infarction from radionuclide activity in the blood pool. The anterior and lateral views of a blood pool scan seen in Figure 10-6, *A* and *B* show radionuclide activity in the entire myocardium. Figure 10-6, *C* and *D* show an anterior wall infarction labeled with ^{99m}Tc PYP. Notice that 10-6*C* could easily be mistaken for a blood

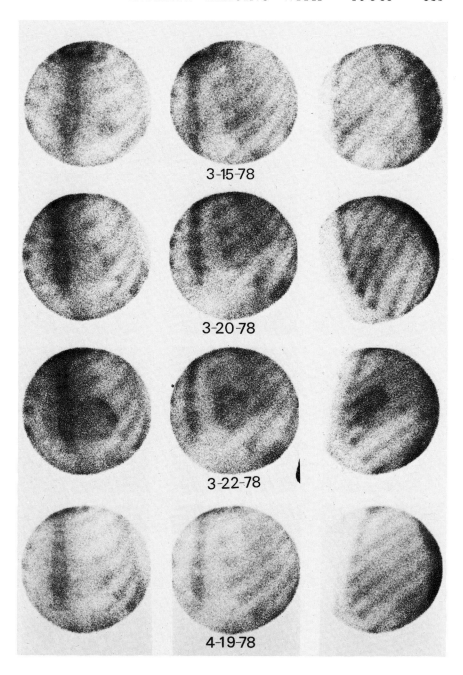

Figure 10-5. Anterior (column 1), left anterior oblique (column 2), and left lateral (column 3) Tc-99m PYP scintigrams in a patient who began with a small anterior apical acute myocardial infarction (first row), extended the infarction to nearly the entire anterior wall (rows 2 and 3), and whose scintigrams reverted back to near normal approximately one month later (row 4). A good example of the need for serial imaging.

BLOOD POOL   INFARCT

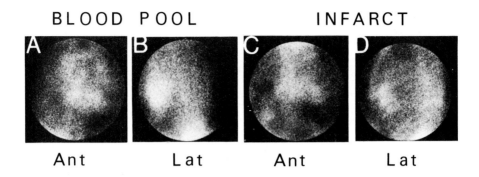

Ant   Lat   Ant   Lat

Figure 10-6. Sequential Tc-99m PYP myocardial scintigrams obtained within minutes (A and B) and over one hour (C and D) after intravenous injection of Tc-99m PYP in the same patient. The blood pool scintigram (A and B) is characterized by a very large and globular area of increased activity in both the anterior (A) and left lateral (B) projections. The true positive myocardial scintigram (C and D) shows relatively diffuse activity in the anterior projection (C) but a relatively localized zone of increased activity along the anterior cardiac surface in the lateral projection.

pool shown in the anterior view only. By using the views in multiple projections, the chances of misinterpreting a blood pool as a false-positive scintigram are decreased.

Different Patterns of Myocardial Uptake

In order to analyze the ^{99m}Tc PYP myocardial scan, it is essential to determine whether the uptake follows one of the recognizable patterns:

1. Well localized—includes doughnut patterns or homogeneous patterns that can be localized to specific myocardial walls, i.e., anterior, lateral, inferior, septal, etc. while using multiple views.

2. Poorly localized—demonstrates activity usually of low intensity, which does not involve the entire myocardium and cannot be localized to a particular region because it is visualized in limited views only.

3. Blood pool activity—includes true blood pool activity resulting from either technical causes, the patient's blood chemistry, or physiology. This group also includes patients with diffuse ^{99m}Tc PYP uptake throughout the myocardium due to metastatic calcification or other conditions that are not yet well defined.

The most common cause of a false positive scan is the misinterpretation of blood pool activity. It is important to realize that if there is a question of blood pool activity, the scintigrams cannot be reliably interpreted and should be repeated after 48 hours.

Grading of the Myocardial Uptake

The scans were graded on a 0 to 4+ positive scale[18] (Fig. 10-7). This scale is entirely arbitrary, but allows comparison of follow-up scans on the basis of intensity of the lesion and not on the basis of size or location of ^{99m}Tc PYP uptake. Zero represents a distinctly negative scan, while the 1+ category was inserted to allow for questionable blood pools, chest wall damage or other activity not associated with the myocardium. Two plus positive (2+) signifies some evidence of activity in the myocardium. Three (3+) and four (4+) plus positive represent increasing amounts of radionuclide activity in the myocardium. Again, it must be pointed out that the degree of activity in the infarcted tissue depends on the blood flow to the injured tissue and the stage when the myocardial imaging was done.

Clinical Usefulness

Three general areas of clinical usefulness for the ^{99m}Tc PYP myocardial scintigraphy are listed below:
1. Diagnosis of acute myocardial infarction
   a. Transmural infarcts
   b. Subendocardial myocardial infarctions
   c. Necrosis in patients with unstable angina pectoris
   d. Extension of myocardial infarction
   e. Perioperative myocardial infarctions
2. Prognosis using serial imaging
3. Sizing acute anterior and anterolateral myocardial infarcts
   a. Help determine prognosis
   b. In the future, to potentially evaluate therapeutic interventions.

Acute Transmural Myocardial Infarcts

Figure 10-8 shows an example of acute transmural myocardial infarction detected by ^{99m}Tc PYP myocardial imaging. At our institution, the

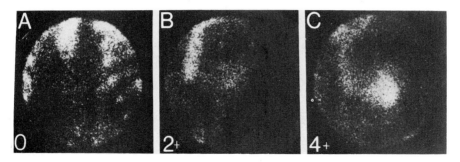

Figure 10-7. Myocardial scintigrams obtained after Tc-99m PYP injection are shown. *A*, Negative myocardial scintigrams; *B*, 2+ activity; *C*, 4+ myocardial uptake of Tc-99m PYP. (Reproduced from Willerson, J.T., et al.: Technetium stannous pyrophosphate myocardial scintigrams in patients with chest pain of varying etiology. *Circulation* **51**: 1047, 1975. Used with permission of the American Heart Association, Inc.)

accuracy in detecting acute transmural myocardial infarcts is greater than 90 percent with serial myocardial imaging of the infarcted region. [23,35-37] In general, the localization of myocardial infarction by ^{99m}Tc imaging correlates well with the localization by electrocardiogram. Sometimes, however, the infarcted regions suggested by ^{99m}Tc PYP uptake are greater than those suggested by electrocardiogram.

Acute Subendocardial Infarcts

In general, we have found that ^{99m}Tc PYP imaging is not as useful in detecting acute infarcts that are nontransmural as for detecting those

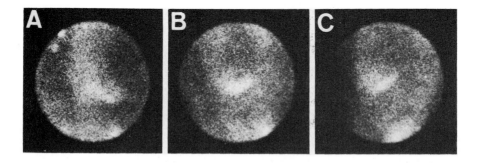

Figure 10-8. Acute inferior myocardial infarct seen on Tc-99m PYP scintigrams in the anterior, left anterior oblique (LAO), and left lateral projections. Note the L-shaped configuration when infarct and sternum combine on the anterior view.

that are transmural, if both are of similar size. Figure 10-9 shows a ^{99m}Tc PYP scintigram of a patient with an abnormality in the inferior wall of the heart and clinical evidence of an inferior subendocardial infarct. However, accuracy of the ^{99m}Tc PYP scintigrams in diagnosing acute subendocardial infarcts varies greatly with different patient populations across the country. This may be due to both the difficulty in making this diagnosis with other modalites and the fact that a large number of these patients have 2+ low-grade positive scans. As the grade or intensity of the scan decreases, the effect of any residual blood pool becomes greater; therefore, quality control is more critical in this group of patients. Some patients have an electrocardiogram which is suggestive of, but not diagnostic of, a subendocardial infarction. The scans can be dramatically positive as in Figure 10-10, possibly as a result of a better collateral flow than generally occurs with this type of infarct.

Unstable Angina Pectoris

In the group of patients with unstable angina pectoris [1,29] approximately one-third have low-grade positive scans as seen in Figure 10-11. Initially, these were believed to represent "false-positive" scintigrams; but histology from some patients revealed microscopic myocardial necrosis in many of these patients [23]. The clinical significance of this finding is not known at this time, but research efforts are underway to evaluate whether patients with unstable angina pectoris and abnormal ^{99m}Tc PYP

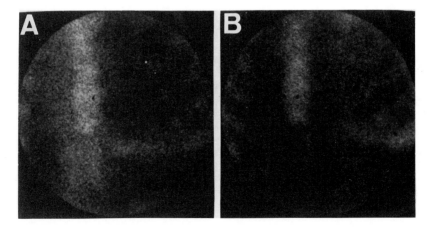

Figure 10-9.   Acute inferior subendocardial myocardial infarct seen on the Tc-99m PYP scintigrams in the anterior and left anterior oblique (LAO) views.

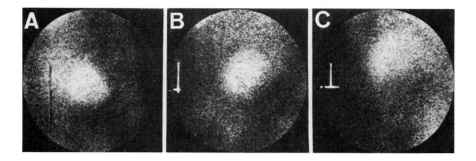

Figure 10-10. 4+ positive Tc-99m PYP scintigrams in the anterior (*A*), LAO (*B*), and left lateral (*C*) views of a patient with the diagnosis of acute subendocardial myocardial infarction by electrocardiogram.

scintigrams have a different clinical course than those with negative scintigrams.

Infarct Extensions and Perioperative Infarction

As demonstrated in Figures 10-5 and 10-12, infarct extension can be diagnosed as an area of increased activity in a new segment of myocardium and/or a wider region of ^{99m}Tc PYP uptake than was initially demonstrated. The ability to identify infarct extension requires new damage of at least 3 grams or more. For detection of small extensions in

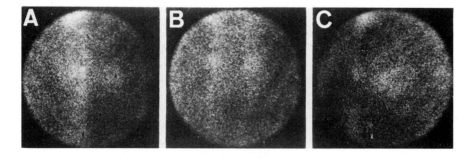

Figure 10-11. Tc-99m PYP myocardial scintigrams in the anterior (*A*), left anterior oblique (*B*), and left lateral (*C*) views in a patient diagnosed as having unstable angina pectoris. This patient's electrocardiogram and enzyme studies were normal while the scintigrams were positive.

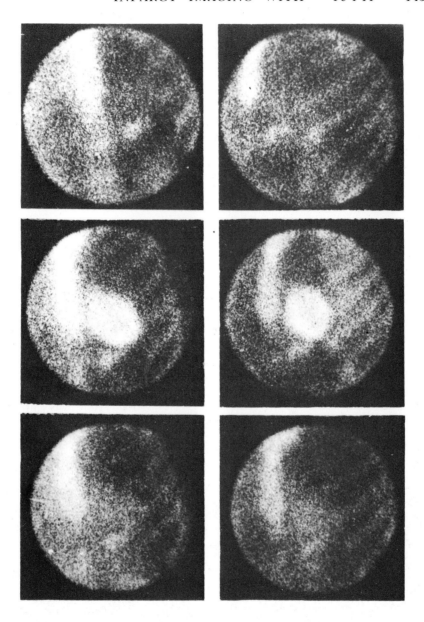

Figure 10-12. Tc-99m PYP myocardial scintigrams in the anterior (left column) and left anterior oblique (right column) showing a patient with extensions of an anterior wall myocardial infarction. Note on the upper panels the small anterior wall myocardial infarction which was diagnosed on electrocardiogram and scintigrams. Approximately two week later, the patient had another onset of severe chest pain and 24 hours after the onset of chest pain, the second row of scintigrams was obtained showing a large area of extension. The lower panel was taken two weeks after the second row and shows marked decreased activity. (Reproduced from Willerson, J.T., et al.: Technetium stannous pyrophosphate myocardial scintigrams in patients with chest pain of varying etiology. *Circulation* **51**: 1050, 1975. Used with permission of the American Heart Association, Inc.)

the same general region of damage, tomographic imaging will probably be required. Also, the use of the technique in identifying perioperative infarctions in which such modalities as enzyme levels and electrocardiograms have limited value, has been well demonstrated.[21,22]

Persistent "Positive" [99m]Tc PYP Scintigrams

Earlier in this chapter we discussed the value of serial imaging with ^{99m}Tc PYP in the diagnosis of acute myocardial infarctions, but we would also like to point out the value of delayed serial imaging in predicting the patient's prognosis (Fig. 10-13). Ours and several other groups including Olsen, et al.[4,17,26] have shown that if a ^{99m}Tc PYP myocardial scintigram is positive three months or longer after the infarction, the patient's prognosis is guarded. In their experience, this group of patients has a higher incidence of cardiac deaths and recurring symptoms including congestive heart failure and severe angina.[17] We believe that still larger numbers of patients need to be evaluated, but if it can be substantiated that those with "persistently abnormal" [99m]Tc PYP myocardial scintigrams have a troubled clinical course, then this imaging technique can be used to provide prognostic information, as well as test various therapeutic interventions.

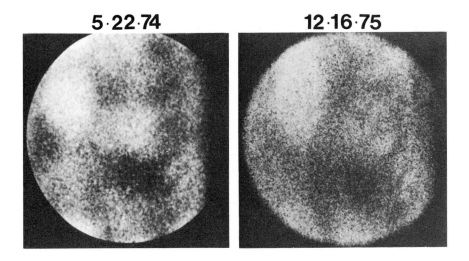

5·22·74   **12·16·75**

Figure 10-13. Anterior Tc-99m PYP scintigrams performed 19 months apart showing a continuing positive area of uptake over the anterior myocardium. The activity has decreased from 4+ to 2+, but has roughly the same configuration.

Sizing Acute Myocardial Infarcts

Coronary artery disease affects pacemaking conduction and/or contractile properties of the heart. The size and location of an infarct determines, in part, how much these functions are affected. The larger the infarct, the more these functions—especially the pumping ability—are altered. Several techniques for evaluating size of myocardial infarction are under study, including the rise of enzyme levels, electrocardiographic surface mapping and myocardial imaging with radionuclides.

We have demonstrated that it is possible to use ^{99m}Tc PYP scintigrams to estimate with some accuracy the size of acute anterior or anterolateral myocardial infarctions in dogs and in humans.[15,16,30,31,38] There is a close correlation between weight of infarct as measured during histologic examination and size of infarct as estimated on a scintigram. At this time, the rate of accuracy is considerably poorer in sizing acute inferior or nontransmural myocardial infarction.

Summary

Presently, the ^{99m}Tc PYP scintigrams are useful in diagnosing acute myocardial necrosis. They may be of value in predicting long-term prognosis and in estimating the size of acute transmural infarctions in the anterior myocardium. These tests, when performed correctly can be valuable to the clinician in evaluating pathophysiological processes in the myocardium when the patient has clinical symptoms of chest pain.

References

1. Alison, H.W., Moraski, R.E., Mantle, J.A., et al.: Coronary anatomy and arteriography in patients with unstable angina pectoris. *Am J Cardiol* **35**:118, 1975 (Abs).
2. Bonte, F.J., Parkey, R.W., Graham, K.D., et al.: A new method for radionuclide imaging of myocardial infarcts. *Radiology* **110**:473-474, 1974.
3. Bruno, F.P., Cobb, F.R., Rivas, F., et al.: Evaluation of ^{99m}technetium-stannous pyrophosphate as an imaging agent in acute myocardial infarction. *Circulation* **54**:71, 1976.
4. Buja, L.M., Poliner, L.R., Parkey, R.W., et al.: Clinicopathologic study of persistently positive technetium-99m stannous pyrophosphate myocardial scintigrams and myocytolytic degeneration after myocardial infarction. *Circulation* **56**:1016-1023, 1977.
5. Buja, L.M., Parkey, R.W., Dees, J.H., et al.: Morphologic correlates of

technetium-99m stannous pyrophosphate imaging of acute myocardial infarcts in dogs. *Circulation* **52**:596-607, 1975.

6. Buja, L.M., Parkey, R.W., Stokely, E.M., et al.: Pathophysiology of technetium-99m stannous pyrophosphate and thallium-201 scintigraphy of acute anterior myocardial infarcts in dogs. *J Clin Invest* **57**:1508-1522, 1976.

7. Buja, L.M., Tofe, A.J., Kulkarni, P.V., et al.: Sites and mechanisms of localization of technetium-99m phosphorus radiopharmaceuticals in acute myocardial infarcts and other tissues. *J Clin Invest* **60**:724-740, 1977.

8. D'Agostino, A.N.: An electron microscopic study of cardiac necrosis produced by 9-α-fluorocortisol and sodium phosphate. *Am J Pathol* **45**:633-644, 1964.

9. Donsky, M.S., Curry, G.C., Parkey, R.W., et al.: Unstable angina pectoris: Clinical, angiographic, and myocardial scintigraphic observations. *Br Heart J* **38**:257-263, 1976.

10. Eliot, R.S., and Edwards, J.E.: Pathology of coronary atherosclerosis and its complications. In Hurst, J.W.(Ed.): *The Heart*, 3rd ed. New York, McGraw-Hill, 1974, p. 1003.

11. Holman, B.L., Lesch, M., Zweiman, F.G., et al.: Detection and sizing of acute myocardial infarcts with [99m]Tc(Sn) tetracycline. *N Engl J Med* **291**: 159-163, 1974.

12. Harford, W., Weinberg, M.N., Buja, L.M., et al.: Positive ^{99m}Tc-stannous pyrophosphate myocardial image in a patient with carcinoma of the lung. *Radiology* **122**:747-748, 1977.

13. Jacobstein, J.G., Alonso, D.R., Roberts, A.J., et al.: Early diagnosis of myocardial infarction in the dog with ^{99m}Tc-glucoheptonate. *J Nucl Med* **18**:413-418, 1977.

14. Khaw, B.A., Beller, G.A., Haber, E., et al.: Localization and sizing of myocardial infarcts employing radioactively labeled myosin specific antibody. *Clin Res* **23**:381A, 1975 (Abs).

15. Lewis, M., Buja, L.M., Saffer, S., et al.: Experimental infarct sizing utilizing three dimensional computer processing reconstruction techniques. *Clin Res* **25**:46A, 1977.

16. Lewis, M., Buja, L.M., Saffer, S., et al.: Experimental infarct sizing using computer processing and a three-dimensional model. *Science* **197**:167-169, 1977.

17. Olson, H., Lyons, K., Aronow, W.S., et al.: Prognostic implications of a persistently positive technetium-99m pyrophosphate myocardial scintigram after acute myocardial infarction. *Clin Res* **26**:96A, Feb 1978.

18. Parkey, R.W., Bonte, F.J., Meyer, S.L., et al.: A new method for radionuclide imaging of acute myocardial infarction in humans. *Circulation* **50**:540-546, 1974.

19. Parkey, R.W., Bonte, F.J., Stokely, E.M., et al.: Acute myocardial infarction imaged with ^{99m}Tc-stannous pyrophosphate and [201]Tl: A clinical evaluation. *J Nucl Med* **17**:771-779, 1976.

20. Perez, L.A.: Clinical experience: Technetium-99m labeled phosphates in

myocardial imaging. *Clin Nucl Med* **1**:2-9, 1976.

21. Platt, M.R., Mills, L.J., Parkey, R.W., et al.: Perioperative myocardial infarction diagnosed by technetium-99m stannous pyrophosphate myocardial scintigrams. *Circulation* **54** (Suppl III):24-27, 1976.

22. Platt, M.R., Parkey, R.W., Willerson, J.T., et al.: Technetium stannous pyrophosphate myocardial scintigrams in the recognition of myocardial infarction in patients undergoing coronary artery revascularization. *Ann Thor Surg* **21**:311-317, 1976.

23. Poliner, L.R., Buja, L.M., Parkey, R.W., et al.: Clinicopathological studies in 52 patients studied with technetium-99m stannous pyrophosphate myocardial scintigraphy. *Circulation*, in press.

24. Poliner, L.R., Buja, L.M., Parkey, R.W., et al.: Comparison of different noninvasive methods of infarct sizing during experimental myocardial infarction. *J Nucl Med* **18**:517-523, 1977.

25. Poliner, L.R., Parkey, R.W., Buja, L.M., et al.: Technetium-99m stannous pyrophosphate myocardial scintigraphy in the recognition of acute subendocardial myocardial infarction. *Texas Med* **73**:74-81, 1977.

26. Poliner, L.R., Hutcheson, D., Buja, L.M., et al.: Persistently positive technetium-99m stannous pyrophosphate myocardial scintigrams after acute myocardial infarction. *Clin Res* **25**:7A, 1977 (Abs).

27. Pugh, B.R., Buja, L.M., Parkey, R.W., et al.: Cardioversion and "false positive" technetium-99m stannous pyrophosphate myocardial scintigrams. *Circulation* **54**:399-403, 1976.

28. Pulido, J.I., Parkey, R.W., Buja, L.M., et al.: Recognition of acute subendocardial myocardial infarcts in patients using technetium-99m stannous pyrophosphate scintigraphy. Submitted 1978.

29. Roberts, W.C.: The coronary arteries and left ventricle in clinically isolated angina pectoris. A necropsy analysis. *Circulation* **54**:388-390, 1976.

30. Rude, R., Parkey, R.W., Bonte, F.J., et al.: Clinical implications of the technetium-99m stannous pyrophosphate myocardial scintigraphic "doughnut" pattern in patients with acute myocardial infarcts. *Circulation*, in press.

31. Stokely, E.M., Buja, L.M., Lewis, S.E., et al.: Measurement of acute myocardial infarcts in dogs with ^{99m}Tc-stannous pyrophosphate scintigrams. *J Nucl Med* **17**:1-5, 1976.

32. Stokely, E.M., Parkey, R.W., Bonte, F.J., et al.: Gated blood pool imaging following ^{99m}Tc-stannous pyrophosphate imaging. *Radiology* **120**:433-434, 1976.

33. Shen, A.C., and Jennings, R.B.: Myocardial calcium and magnesium in acute ischemic injury. *Am J Pathol* **67**:417-440, 1972.

34. Willerson, J.T., Parkey, R.W., Bonte, F.J., et al.: Acute subendocardial myocardial infarction in patients. Its detection by technetium-99m stannous pyrophosphate myocardial scintigrams. *Circulation* **51**:436-441, 1975.

35. Willerson, J.T., Parkey, R.W., Bonte, F.J., et al.: Technetium stannous pyrophosphate myocardial scintigrams in patients with chest pain of vary-

ing etiology. *Circulation* **51**:1046-1052, 1975.

36. Willerson, J.T., Parkey, R.W., Bonte, F.J., et al.: Technetium stannous pyrophosphate myocardial scintigraphy for diagnosing and localizing acute myocardial infarcts. *Texas Med* **72**:61, 1976.

37. Willerson, J.T., Parkey, R.W., Buja, L.M., et al.: Are ^{99m}Tc-stannous pyrophosphate myocardial scintigrams clinically useful? *Clin Nucl Med* **2**:137-145, 1977 (editorial).

38. Willerson, J.T., Parkey, R.W., Stokely, E.M., et al.: Infarct sizing with technetium-99m stannous pyrophosphate scintigraphy in dogs and man; relationship between scintigraphic and precordial mapping estimates of infarct size in patients. *Cardiovasc Res* **11**:291-298, 1977.

39. Zaret, B.L., DiCola, V.C., Donabedian, R.K., et al.: Dual radionuclide study of myocardial infarction. Relationships between myocardial uptake of potassium-43, technetium-99m stannous pyrophosphate, regional myocardial blood flow and creatine phosphokinase depletion. *Circulation* **53**:422-428, 1976.

CHAPTER XI

Acute Myocardial Infarction Imaging with Thallium-201

Jagmeet S. Soin, M.D., and Harold L. Brooks, M.D.

The value and limitations of the infarct-avid (technetium-99m pyrophosphate) myocardial imaging agents have been pointed out by Parkey et al. in the preceding chapter. The myocardial perfusion dependent agents such as thallium-201 chloride can also be used to evaluate acute myocardial infarction. When seeking an ideal agent for imaging acute myocardial infarctions the following questions must be considered: (1) Is the technique sufficiently sensitive and specific for the detection of acute myocardial infarction? (2) How soon can an accurate diagnosis be made after the onset of clinical symptoms? (3) How accurately can the site of infarction be determined? (4) Can the size of myocardial infarction be determined accurately? (5) What is the cost and availability of the test? Answers to these questions reveal that both techniques complement each other in the evaluation of a patient who is either suspected of having or who already has an acute myocardial infarction.

The thallium-201 myocardial perfusion study is performed at the bedside in a patient who is suspected of having an acute myocardial infarction. This limits the means to reduce the background activity in the splanchnic blood pool. Whenever possible, this test should be performed after three to four hours of fasting and the injection should be made with the patient sitting upright in order to reduce the splanchnic blood pool activity. A portable scintillation camera is necessary to perform studies at the bedside. Several excellent commercial models are now available. A detailed consideration of portable imaging devices is made in Chapter 20. The gamma camera is equipped with a high resolution collimator. Multiple images of the myocardium are obtained 20 minutes after injection. The thallium-201 myocardial scintigram can be recognized by increased background activity and absence of radioactivity in the right ventricular myocardium. A normal thallium study done in a patient suspected of acute myocardial infarction is shown in Figure 11-1.

In documenting the sensitivity of thallium-201 myocardial perfusion imaging in acute myocardial infarction, Wackers et al. reported that of 200 patients with documented myocardial infarctions, 82 percent showed definite perfusion abnormalities on myocardial scintigrams. This is similar to the overall sensitivity for ^{99m}Tc (Sn) pyrophosphate in the detection of acute transmural infarction. However, two factors influence the accuracy of thallium myocardial perfusion studies: (1) time elapsed between the onset of symptoms and the time the study is performed, and (2) the site and size of the infarction. A thallium study is more accurate for detecting myocardial infarction within 8 hours after the onset of symptoms than it is later in the clinical course. If the detection of acute myocardial ischemia has to be documented within 18 hours after the onset of symptoms, ^{201}Tl scintigraphy may be the preferred study, since uptake of ^{99m}Tc-pyrophosphate is seldom evident before 18 hours after the onset of symptoms. Although the thallium-201 study is quite sensitive in deteting a myocardial perfusion defect, it is not nearly as specific for detecting an acute myocardial infarction as is technetium pyrophosphate. A well known limitation of all monovalent cations used in myocardial perfusion imaging is that they do not allow distinction between areas of acute ischemia and recent or old myocardial infarction. However, on the other hand, in an uncomplicated myocardial infarction, uptake of ^{99m}Tc-pyrophosphate is seldom seen by the third week fol-

Tl-201 Myocardial Perfusion Study at Rest

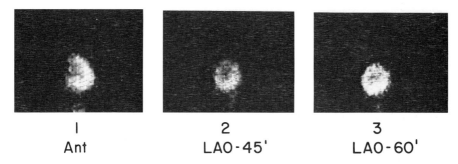

| 1 | 2 | 3 |
| Ant | LAO-45' | LAO-60' |

Figure 11-1. Thallium-201 myocardial perfusion study with patient at rest in anterior, LAO 45°, and LAO 60° views. Note the uniform distributions of radioactivity in the left ventricle. No activity is seen in the right ventricle. Note the normal areas of decreased radioactivity in the upper portion of the interventricular septum and aortic root.

lowing an acute episode. In contrast, a thallium-201 myocardial perfusion study can remain abnormal indefinitely; thus, it is a preferred test if the possibility of remote myocardial infarction is to be evaluated. Certainly then it is not surprising that thallium-201 myocardial perfusion and ^{99m}Tc-pyrophosphate studies are complementary and an accuracy rate of 100 percent has been demonstrated by Berger et al. when both studies are used together to detect acute myocardial infarction.[3]

In determining the site of acute myocardial infarction, thallium-201 scintigraphy may be slightly more accurate than a technetium-99m pyrophosphate scan. Since thallium-201 accumulates in a normal myocardium, it provides a way of localizing the perfusion defects. Technetium-99m pyrophosphate, on the other hand, only accumulates in the abnormal tissue and provides no reference for normal myocardial tissue, thus making the exact localization of infarction somewhat more difficult. In a clinicopathological study, Wackers et al. demonstrated that the location of acute myocardial infarction in the anterior and inferior wall could be predicted on thallium-201 scintigraphy with reasonable accuracy.[2] However, difficulty arose in detecting posterior wall myocardial infarctions. The relative accuracy of technetium-99m pyrophosphate and thallium-201 in detecting the site of infarction has not been studied in detail; however, Berger and colleagues have also shown slightly greater accuracy for predicting the site of infarction on thallium-201 studies than on technetium-99m pyrophosphate scans.[3]

Both of these myocardial imaging agents are of limited value in predicting accurate size of the myocardial infarction. In a population of patients with documented acute myocardial infarctions, larger infarct sizes were predicted on technetium-99m pyrophosphate studies than on thallium-201 images. Overestimation of size was less common in thallium-201 studies.[3] A look at pathophysiology may help explain this difference. Experimental studies demonstrate linear relationships between thallium distribution and both regional myocardial blood flow and depletion of creatine phosphokinase.[4,5] In contrast, uptake of technetium-99m pyrophosphate is not related directly to regional blood flow or creatine phosphokinase depletion.[4] A decrease in technetium-99m pyrophosphate is noted when the coronary blood flow is reduced to 30 to 40 percent below normal. In peripheral areas of relatively good flow, significant accumulation of technetium-99m pyrophosphate can be seen.[6] No simple relationship has been found between the extent of necrosis and degree of pyrophosphate uptake. The combination of increased uptake in a border zone and variable uptake in a necrosed tissue as seen on a technetium-99m pyrophosphate scan may lead to overestimation of infarct size.[7] However, Parkey and associates have found contradictory results suggesting that thallium-201 overestimates the size of infarction.[8] A case of apparent discrepancy in two studies is demonstrated in Figure 11-2. Neither of the two agents are expected to provide reliable estimation of infarct size because neither is helpful in detecting small infarctions.

A resulting thallium-201 image may be useful in early screening of patients admitted to coronary care units for suspected acute myocardial infarction because of its high sensitivity in the detection of regions of decreased myocardial perfusion. In a study of selected patients who had atypical chest pain or nondiagnostic abnormalities on electrocardiograms, an abnormal thallium scintigram was found to be a good indicator of infarction. Patients in this study who had normal thallium-201 scintillation studies on admission did not develop acute myocardial infarction on follow-up. These findings suggest that thallium-201 may

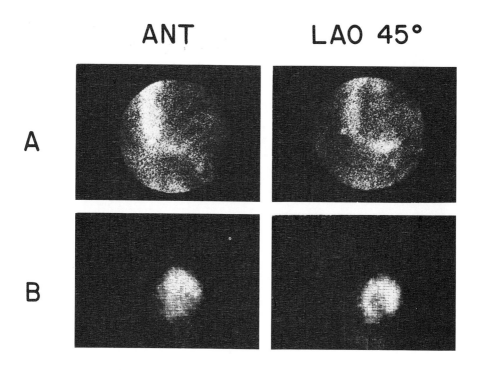

Figure 11-2.   *A,* Technetium-99m pyrophosphate scan in a patient with acute inferior myocardial infarction. *B,* Thallium-201 study in the same patient. These figures highlight the difficulty in assessing the size of myocardial infarction. In the LAO 45° view the area of technetium-99m pyrophosphate uptake appears larger than the defect seen on the thallium-201 study.

play a role in triaging patients intended for cardiac care units.[9]

In summary, in the proper clinical setting, thallium-201 scintigraphy can be useful in the following three circumstances: (1) for detecting acute myocardial infarction within 18 hours after the onset of symptoms, (2) for triaging patients admitted to cardiac care units, and (3) for detecting remote myocardial infarction. A thallium-201 study is somewhat more accurate than a technetium-99m pyrophosphate study for determining the site of an infarction; however, neither of the techniques seems accurate in determining the size of myocardial infarction. In the final analysis, the current cost and availability of thallium-201 chloride may prevent its use in the community hospital; however, these factors may change in the near future.

References

1. Wackers, F.J., Sokole, E.B., Samson, G., et al.:   Value and limitation of thallium-201 scintigraphy in the acute phase of myocardial infarction.   *N Engl J Med* **295**:1-15, 1976.

2. Wackers, F.J., TH., Becker, A.E., Sampson, G., et al.:   Location and size of acute myocardial infarction predicted by thallium-201 scintiscans—clinicopathological correlation. *Circulation* **56**:72-78, 1977.

3. Berger, H.J., Gottschalk, A., and Zaret, B.L.:   Dual radionuclide study of acute myocardial infarction. *Ann Int Med* **88**:145-154, 1978.

4. Zaret, B.L., Dicola, V.C., Donabedian, R.K., et al.:   Dual radionuclide study of myocardial infarction.   Relationship between myocardial uptake of K-43, Tc-99m (Sn) PYP, regional blood flow and creatine phosphokinase depletion. *Circulation* **53**:422-428, 1976.

5. Dicola, V.C., Downing, S.E., Donabedian, R.K., et al.:   Pathophysiological correlates of thallium-201 uptake in experimental infarction. *Cardiovasc Res* **11**:141-146, 1977.

6. Buja, L.M., Parkey, R.W., Dees, J.H., et al.:   Morphological correlates of Tc-99m stannous pyrophosphate imaging of acute myocardial infarcts in dogs. *Ciculation* **52**:596-607, 1975.

7. Zaret, B.L., Lange, R., and Lee, J.:   Comparative assessment of infarct size with quantitative thallium-201 and Tc-99m pyrophosphate dual myocardial infarct imaging in the dog (Abs). *Am J Card* **31**:308, 1977.

8. Parkey, R.W., Bonte, F.J., Stokley, E.M., et al.:   Acute myocardial infarction imaged with Tc-99m stannous pyrophosphate and Tl-201—A clinical evaluation. *J Nucl Med* **17**:771-779, 1976.

9. Wackers, F.J., Lie, K.I., Sokole, E.B., et al.:   Prospective study of the value of thallium-201 scinitgraphy for selection of CCU patients. *Circulation* **53** (II):848, 1976 (Abstract).

CHAPTER XII

Diffuse Pattern of [99m]Tc Pyrophosphate Myocardial Uptake: A Dilemma

Masood Ahmad, M.D., and Jagmeet S. Soin, M.D.

Technetium-99m pyrophosphate myocardial imaging is being used widely to diagnose acute myocardial infarction.[1,2] Since its introduction in clinical medicine, several studies have been performed to evaluate the sensitivity and specificity of ^{99m}Tc pyrophosphate myocardial imaging in the detection of acute myocardial infarction.[3,7] At the present time, this technique seems most useful in diagnosing acute myocardial infarction when the traditional means of diagnosis, i.e., electrocardiogram and serum enzyme changes, are inadequate. However, one of the major problems in the evaluation of ^{99m}Tc PYP myocardial scan is that approximately 16 percent of cardiac patients and 13 percent of noncardiac patients show radioactivity in the cardiac region which has a diffuse pattern.[7] Thus in any assessment of ^{99m}Tc-PYP myocardial imaging, a consideration of the factors responsible for nonfocal (diffuse) cardiac uptake in the patient suffering from cardiac or noncardiac illness is quite important.

To understand the clinical implications of the diffuse pattern of ^{99m}Tc pyrophosphate myocardial scintigram, it is important to be familiar with the image interpretation process.

Image Interpretation

A ^{99m}Tc pyrophosphate myocardial scintigram may be evaluated for (1) intensity of concentration of the radionuclide in the myocardium, (2) pattern of distribution of radionuclide in the myocardium, and (3) area of the myocardium where the radionuclide has concentrated. Parkey et al. have graded the intensity of uptake from zero to 4+. Zero represents no activity; 1+ indicates definite myocardial activity and should be read as negative; 2+ indicates definite myocardial activity but not equal to sternal activity; 3+ refers to activity equal to sternal uptake; and 4+ activity greater than sternal uptake. The pattern of uptake may be classified as "focal" when the uptake is discrete, "diffuse" when the edges of the uptake are poorly defined, and as "doughnut pattern" when the uptake is in the form of a large rim with a clear central zone.

Sensitivity and Specificity of ^{99m}Tc PYP Myocardial Imaging

The issue of sensitivity and specificity of this technique in the diagnosis of acute myocardial infarction is somewhat controversial. Histologic studies have demonstrated that infarcts weighing less than three grams have not been identified even with serial imaging.[8,9] Thus small areas of myocardial necrosis may not be detectable by this technique. The clinical significance of such small areas of myocardial infarction, not detectable by presently available techniques, is not known. The initial reports concerning the specificity of a positive ^{99m}Tc pyrophosphate myocardial scintigram were overly optimistic. In our experience the "doughnut" pattern of uptake is most specific for acute myocardial infarction. A focal pattern is also highly specific for acute myocardial infarction if a ventricular aneurysm can be excluded. The least specific is the diffuse pattern of myocardial uptake.

Does the diffuse uptake result from subclinical myocardial necrosis undetectable by electrocardiogram and enzyme levels in the blood or does it represent a technical error? This question may be difficult to answer in a given patient. To limit the likelihood of technical errors, it is important to: (1) make certain that the ^{99m}Tc pyrophosphate injectant does not contain an excess of free technetium-99m pertechnetate (an excess could result in labeling of red blood cells so that the cardiac pool shows up on the scintigrams). (2) Begin imaging at least 1.5 to 2 hours after the ^{99m}Tc pyrophosphate injection. This will avoid the problem of imaging the intracardiac blood pool activity. (3) Exercise caution when interpreting scintigrams of patients with impaired renal function and/or low cardiac ouput. In these patients the radionuclide clears the blood pool more slowly, creating a diffuse pattern on the ^{99m}Tc pyrophosphate scintigram. In order to evaluate its clinical significance, only diffuse cardiac uptake of 2+ or more is considered important. As indicated earlier, any cardiac uptake of a lesser degree is generally related to cardiac blood pool activity. Recently described computerized methods utilizing subtraction techniques may also aid in separating true from false positive scans.[10]

The Diffuse Pattern

To evaluate the specificity of ^{99m}Tc pyrophosphate myocardial imaging in clinical diagnosis, we studied 67 patients with clinically apparent heart disease, but without myocardial infarction. Diffuse patterns of ^{99m}Tc pyrophosphate uptake as shown in Figure 12-1 was seen in seven of 30 patients with stable angina pectoris, three of three patients with unstable angina pectoris, four of thirteen patients who had aortocoronary bypass surgery, four of four patients with congestive cardiomyopathy and in one patient who had cardioversion the day before the study. In 14 of these patients (73 percent) with diffuse patterns, the intensity of the concentration of radionuclide was 3+.[4] Our observations of positive scintigrams in patients with stable and unstable angina pectoris have been confirmed by others.[11,12] But several other reports further highlight the dilemma: Uptake of ^{99m}Tc pyrophosphate in the myocardium may also occur in some patients who have had myocardial infarction in the past,[13] valve calcification,[14] myocardial or adjacent neoplasm,[15] and radiation therapy of the chest.[16] Table 12-1 lists the various conditions in which the diffuse pattern of ^{99m}Tc pyrophosphate myocardial uptake may be found.

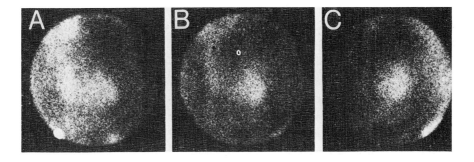

Figure 12-1. Diffuse pattern of ^{99m}Tc pyrophosphate myocardial uptake in a patient with acute nontransmural myocardial infarction shown in the anterior (*A*), left anterior oblique (*B*), and left lateral views (*C*).

TABLE 12-1
Conditions Associated with Diffuse Pattern of Tc-99m Pyrophosphate
Myocardial Uptake

1.	Acute myocardial infarction	6.	Cardiac or adjacent neoplasm
	Transmural	7.	Congestive cardiomyopathy
	Nontransmural (subendocardial)	8.	Left ventricular aneurysm
2.	Unstable angina pectoris	9.	Calcified cardiac valves
3.	Previous myocardial infarction	10.	Stable angina pectoris
4.	Post D.C. cardioversion	11.	Post chest irradiation
5.	Cardiac trauma	12.	Unexplained conditions

Predictive Value of the Diffuse Pattern

Present literature is relatively scant with respect to definitive studies. We have addressed the issue of predictability of acute necrosis by the diffuse pattern.

Angina Pectoris

We followed a group of 26 patients with stable angina pectoris for a period of two years.[17] Five of these 26 patients had scans with diffuse patterns of ^{99m}Tc pyrophosphate myocardial uptake and no clinical evidence of acute myocardial infarction. There was no significant difference in the incidence of unstable angina pectoris, myocardial infarction or left ventricular failure between patients with and without the diffuse pattern of ^{99m}Tc pyrophosphate uptake. The clinical functional class, severity and frequency of angina, response to nitrates, and electrocardiograms in these five patients were similar in both groups of patients. This data suggests that the presence of a positive technetium-99m pyrophosphate myocardial scintigram in a patient with stable angina pectoris has no apparent diagnostic or prognostic significance. However, these numbers are too small to make any definitive conclusions regarding the pathophysiology of diffuse uptake in patients with angina pectoris.

Acute Myocardial Infarction

To determine the prognostic value of the pattern of technetium-99m pyrophosphate myocardial uptake, we followed 30 survivors of acute myocardial infarction with 3+ or 4+ positive scintigrams. Eight patients with transmural myocardial infarction had a "doughnut" pattern of uptake and sixteen patients had a focal uptake (anterior in seven patients, lateral in two patients, posterior in three patients, and inferior in four patients). All patients with the doughnut pattern of uptake developed late complications of acute myocardial infarction; 68 percent of the patients with scans showing focal patterns developed complications, as did 12 percent of the patients with the diffuse patterns. All patients with the diffuse pattern survived the follow-up period. The mortality rate in the group with scans showing focal patterns was 6 percent, and was 83 percent in the group with scans showing the "doughnut" patterns. These data suggest a favorable long-term prognosis in patients whose scans show the diffuse pattern of uptake. However, caution is suggested in separating blood pool activity from true diffuse myocardial uptake. The reasons for improved prognosis in patients with diffuse uptake is not clear. [18,19]

Until definitive long-term follow-up studies and histologic data become available, the clinical significance of a diffuse pattern of technetium-99m pyrophosphate on myocardial scintigram in patients without other evidence of acute myocardial infarction will continue to be a diagnostic dilemma. However, under appropriate clinical circumstances the presence of significant ^{99m}Tc pyrophosphate activity in the cardiac region is a sensitive indicator for the presence of acute myocardial necrosis, regardless of the pattern of uptake. However, every caution must be taken to distinguish cardiac blood pool activity from significant myocardial uptake.[20] A recent study has demonstrated that a repeat delayed image obtained four hours after injection can distinguish between the activity related to cardiac blood pool or myocardial infarction.[21] The cause of diffuse cardiac uptake seen in noncardiac patients as summarized in Table 12-1 is also unexplained at this time, suggesting the need of thorough clinical evaluation before interpreting the ^{99m}Tc pyrophosphate myocardial scan showing a diffuse pattern of radioactivity.

Acknowledgement

The author is grateful to Dr. Richard H. Martin, Director, Division of Cardiology, University of Missouri Medical Center, for his critical review of this manuscript.

References

1. Bonte, F.J., Parkey, R.W., Graham, K.D., et al.: A new method for radionuclide imaging of myocardial infarcts. *Radiology* 110:473-474, 1974.

2. Parkey, R.W., Bonte, F.J., Meyer, S.L., et al.: A new method for radio-nuclide imaging of acute myocardial infarction in humans. *Circulation* **50**:540-546, 1975.

3. Ahmad, M., Dubiel, J.P., Verdon, T.A., et al.: Technetium-99m stannous pyrophosphate myocardial imaging in patients with and without left ventricular aneurysm. *Circulation* **53**:833-838, 1976.

4. Ahmad, M., Dubiel, J.P., Logan, K.W., et al.: Limited clinical diagnostic specificity of technetium-99m stannous pyrophosphate myocardial imaging in acute myocardial infarction. *Am J Cardiol* **39**:50-54, 1977.

5. Ahmad, M.: Sensitivity and specificity of Tc-99m pyrophosphate myocardial imaging in acute myocardial infarction. *Am J Cardiol* **41**:349, 1978.

6. Cowley, M.J., Mantle, J.A., Rogers, W.J., et al.: Technetium-99m stannous pyrophosphate myocardial scintigraphy: Reliability and limitations in assessment of acute myocardial infarction. *Circulation* **56**:192-198, 1977.

7. Prasquier, R., Taradash, M.R., Botvinick, E.H., et al.: The specificity of the diffuse pattern of cardiac uptake in myocardial infarction imaging with technetium-99m stannous pyrophosphate. *Circulation* **55**:61-65, 1977.

8. Stokely, E.M., Buja, L.M., Lewis, S.E., et al.: Measurement of acute myocardial infarcts in dogs with 99mTc-stannous pyrophosphate scintigrams. *J Nucl Med* **17**:1-5, 1976.

9. Poliner, L.R., Buja, L.M., Parkey, R.W., et al.: Comparison of different noninvasive methods in infarct sizing during experimental myocardial infarction. *J Nucl Med* **18**:523-527, 1977.

10. Berman, D.S., Amsterdam, E.A., Hines, H.H., et al.: Problem of diffuse cardiac uptake of technetium-99m pyrophosphate in the diagnosis of acute myocardial infarction: Enhanced scintigraphic accuracy by computerized selective blood pool subtraction. *Am J Cardiol* **40**:768-774, 1977.

11. Donsky, M.S., Curry, G.C., Parkey, R.W., et al.: Unstable angina pectoris: Clinical angiographic and myocardial scintigraphic observations. *Br Heart J* **38**:257-263, 1976.

12. Mason, J.W., Myers, R.W., Alderman, E.L., et al.: Technetium-99m pyrophosphate myocardial uptake in patients with stable angina pectoris. *Am J Cardiol* **40**:1-5, 1977.

13. Olson, H.G., Lyons, K.P., Arrow, W.S., et al.: Follow-up technetium-99m stannous pyrophosphate myocardial scintigrams after acute myocardial infarction. *Circulation* **56**:181-187, 1977.

14. Joe, S.H., Mean, I., Jengo, J.A., et al.: False positive myocardial infarction scanning: Calcified aortic and mitral valves. Northern and Southern California Chapters, Society of Nuclear Medicine, Los Angeles, California, 1975.

15. Soin, J.S., Burdine, J.A., and Beal, W.: Myocardial localization of 99mTc-pyrophosphate without evidence of acute myocardial infarction. *J Nucl Med* **16**:944-946, 1975.

16. Soin, J.S., Cox, J.D., Youker, J.E., et al.: Cardiac localization of Tc-99m (Sn) pyrophosphate following irradiation of the chest. *Radiology* **124**:165-168, 1977.

17. Ahmad, M., and Martin, R.H.: Technetium-99m stannous pyrophosphate myocardial imaging in patients with stable angina pectoris: A follow-up study. *Clin Res* **25**:201A, 1977 (Abstract).

18. Willerson, J.T., Parkey, R.W., and Bonte, F.J.: Technetium stannous pyrophosphate myocardial scintigrams in patients with chest pain of varying etiology. *Circulation* **51**:1046-1052, 1975.

19. Ahmad, M., Logan, K.W., and Martin, R.H.: Prognostic value of positive Tc-99m pyrophosphate scintigrams in patients with acute myocardial infarction. *Am J Cardiol* **41**:440, 1978 (Abstract).

20. Poliner, L.R., Buja, L.M., Parkey, R.W., et al.: Clinicopathologic findings in 52 patients studied by technetium-99m stannous pyrophosphate myocardial scintigraphy. *Circulation* **59**:257-267, 1979.

21. Cowley, M.J., Mantle, J.A., Rogers, W.J., et al.: Use of blood pool imaging in evaluation of diffuse activity patterns in technetium-99m pyrophosphate myocardial scintigraphy. *J Nucl Med* **20**:496-501, 1979.

CHAPTER XIII

Radionuclide Techniques in the Assessment of Left Ventricular Function: Technical Considerations

James H. Thrall, M.D.
Bertram Pitt, M.D.
Thomas J. Brady, M.D.

Analysis of left ventricular function plays an integral part in the diagnosis and management of many patients with heart disease. Prognosis is often directly influenced by the degree of functional impairment, and serial evaluation of left ventricular function allows documentation of response to therapeutic interventions. Over the past 25 years methods for extracting and quantitating data concerning left ventricular function from contrast ventriculograms have been under intensive development, and a number of diagnostic systems have been proposed for analyzing both global and regional ventricular function.[1] While cardiac catheterization provides much useful information and is the accepted standard against which newer techniques must be validated, the invasiveness and expense of the procedure necessarily limit its clinical use to larger medical centers with specialized catheterization laboratories. These limitations have strongly motivated interest in alternative, less invasive and simpler procedures for evaluating left ventricular function including radionuclide techniques.

One of the earliest applications of radiotracers in clinical medicine was the precordial time-activity recording of radioisotope transit through the central circulation (radiocardiography).[2] Radiocardiography provides information on mean pulmonary and cardiac transit times. Attempts were made to establish diagnostic criteria for congestive heart failure and detection of intracardiac shunts. Although the technique of radiocardiography as originally proposed was never widely used clinically, in many respects the nuclear cardiological procedures available today are simply progressively sophisticated modifications of the original concept.

In 1969 Mullins and co-workers reported an experimental technique for determining ventricular volume and ejection fraction. With this technique a gamma camera was used to record on videotape the first transit of a radioactive bolus injected directly into the left ventricle.[3] Mullins' experimental work on dogs was followed by the report of Strauss and co-workers in 1971 who successfully measured the left ventricular ejection fraction in man using a dual gated equilibrium blood pool technique.[4] The correlation between ejection fraction calculated by the radionuclide technique and contrast ventriculography was good. In the years following these reports, numerous other investigators have confirmed the validity of both approaches while adding useful modifications to the original procedures. The modifications have included development of new instrumentation, alternative data acquisition techniques, calculation of additional parameters of left ventricular function and perhaps most importantly, the use of computers to both control sophisticated data collection routines and to assist in data analysis and display.[5-12]

As the tracer techniques have improved, their acceptance in clinical practice has steadily increased, and radionuclide ventriculography has been applied to an ever widening spectrum of clinical problems. Any discussion of radionuclide ventriculography and left ventricular function analysis will rapidly become out of date, and it would be impossible to describe every technique either proposed or in current use. For example, there are over a dozen nuclear medicine computer systems available commercially, each with unique characteristics. Nonetheless, the fundamental principles underlying radionuclide ventriculography are now quite well established. A thorough grasp of these principles as they apply to data collection and analysis techniques is needed to understand current clinical applications and new technical developments.

Data Collection Techniques
in Radionuclide Ventriculography

The two fundamentally different approaches to data collection described in the report of Mullins[3] and Strauss[4] are both in use clinically. In the "first pass" or "first transit" technique the initial passage of a radiotracer through the heart is monitored by a gamma scintillation camera. The "equilibrium blood pool" technique is performed after an intravascular radiotracer has reached equilibrium and relies on synchronizing data collection intervals with specified portions of the cardiac cycle.

Although the information attainable from the two techniques is largely identical, the requirements such as radiopharmaceuticals, imaging equipment, computers and imaging positions are quite different. The two techniques will be discussed separately and then briefly compared.

First Transit Techniques

Any of several radiopharmaceuticals may be selected for first transit radionuclide ventriculography. If only a single examination is anticipated, any radiotracer such as technetium-99m pertechnetate, which does not diffuse out of the vascular space during its passage through the lungs, could be used. If multiple studies must be done during a short time interval to assess changes in ventricular function, radiopharmaceuticals such as technetium-99m DTPA (diethylenetriamine pentaacetic acid) which is cleared rapidly through the kidneys, or technetium-99m sulfur colloid, which is taken up by the liver, may be preferred. These tracers clear quickly from the blood stream resulting in lower background radioactivity for subsequent studies. Some centers have used a preparation with a high specific concentration of technetium-99m pyrophosphate when ventricular function is being assessed in a patient with suspected myocardial infarction. This allows the initial functional evaluation to be followed by infarct avid imaging.

When multiple studies are done, the dosage of radioactivity must be divided appropriately to limit the total radiation exposure to the patient. In some states there is also a limitation on the amount of radioactivity permissible for outpatient examinations. This restriction must be taken into consideration when determining the amount of radionuclide for each injection and the number of injections.

For first transit studies, satisfactory intravenous bolus injections are necessary to insure proper visualization of the left ventricle without excessive trailing activity in the right heart or the lungs. Satisfactory bolus injections are easiest to obtain with central venous catheters, but in practice this has not been necessary. In a currently accepted approach, a small volume, high specific concentration radiotracer (10 to 25 millicuries in less than 1 ml) is injected rapidly and followed immediately by a 10 to 20 ml saline flush. This technique creates a significantly shorter and more compact bolus than does the Oldendorf technique, which is no longer recommended.[13] If a medial vein is chosen for injections in the antecubital fossa, fragmentation of the bolus between the basilar and cephalic systems is minimized.[14] Hyperextension of the arm and the Valsalva maneuver both cause the tracer to stay at the thoracic inlet and are, therefore, avoided.

The most commonly used camera position for first transit studies is the 20-30° right anterior oblique position. This view provides good separation of the left ventricle from the left atrium, allows delineation of the aortic valve plane and has the added advantage of being a standard projection for comparison with the contrast ventriculography. This facilitates correlations between the nuclear and x-ray procedures, particularly in analyzing regional wall motion. Anterior, left lateral and left posterior oblique positions have also been used, and some centers routinely take both the right anterior oblique and left anterior oblique views.

In early applications of the first pass technique, videotape was used to record the raw data.[3,5,9] Computers are now used for this purpose, and the data are stored in either list mode or frame mode format (see Chapter 4). Data collection is started before the bolus reaches the left ventricle and is continued for 20 to 30 seconds to insure that all the data are recorded. Data may also be collected from the right side of the heart using the same technique by simply initiating the acquisition process before the bolus reaches the right atrium.

The limited time available for data collection during first transit studies places a premium on the sensitivity of the recording device. The high count rate capability of multi-crystal gamma cameras is a recognized advantage of this type of instrument over the single crystal gamma camera for first pass studies. Maximum observed count rates with multi-crystal detectors can exceed 250,000 counts per second with a 10 to 15 millicurie injection.[15]

Even with high sensitivity collimation, the upper limit for current generation single crystal cameras is approximately 80-100,000 counts per second.[17] Nonetheless, first transit studies have been successfully accomplished with Anger type cameras.[3,5,9,11,18,19]

A third alternative instrument for first transit studies is the gamma scintillation probe. The probe technique does not provide images of the cardiac chambers but does provide basic quantitative data for assessing global left ventricular function. In addition to costing substantially less than the multi-crystal or single-crystal gamma cameras, the major advantages of probes are their simplicity and portability. Also smaller amounts of radiotracer are required for probe studies than for the gamma camera based techniques, thereby allowing more frequent serial analysis.[20–22] The major disadvantage of the probe for first pass studies is lack of a method for exactly positioning and repositioning the device with respect to the left ventricle. A second shortcoming of the probe system is the fixed field of view—since the system is based on estimates of average heart size, it may not give accurate results in the face of significant cardiomegaly.[22]

Equilibrium Gated Blood Pool Techniques

Equilibrium blood pool imaging is the alternative to first pass data collection. Choice of radiopharmaceutical is limited to those tracers which remain within the vascular space. In the original gated blood pool technique, 10 to 20 millicuries of technetium-99m human serum albumin was injected intravenously.[4] Although it provides satisfactory results, albumin leaks from the vascular space steadily with time, and due to denaturation of albumin during the radiolabelling process, a significant percentage localizes in the liver. The vascular leakage causes a steady increase in background radioactivity and the hepatic uptake reduces the amount of radioactivity available for heart chamber visualization. More recently, technetium-99m has been used to label red blood cells (see Chapter 3). This may be done either in vitro[23-25] or in vivo by first injecting "cold" stannous pyrophosphate followed 15 to 30 minutes later by a second injection of sodium pertechnetate.[26,27] Both the in vitro and in vivo technetium-99m red blood cell preparations have target-to-background ratios far superior to those of technetium-99m human serum albumin.[29,30] Moreover, repeated imaging is feasible for as long as the count rate is sufficient. With ^{99m}Tc RBC preparations, the limiting factor is the half-life of the radiolabel and not the localization properties of the tracer. In our laboratory, we have successfully imaged the cardiac blood pool as long as 24 hours after labeled red cells were administered. There are no special requirements for injecting the tracer in equilibrium gated blood pool imaging. With routine intravenous techniques, the tracer is injected and allowed to equilibrate for 3 to 5 minutes throughout the vascular space prior to imaging. If the in vivo labeling procedure is used for red blood cells, injection through heparinized catheters reduces the labeling efficiency and is avoided.[29]

A variety of protocols are in current use for equilibrium blood pool imaging. All rely on physiologic signals to identify the phases of the cardiac cycle and to control the time intervals during which scintillation data is obtained (Fig. 13-1). In the original description by Strauss, gated images were taken at end systole and end diastole. The gating "window" for end diastole was taken 60 milliseconds immediately preceeding the R wave. For end systole, data were recorded during the last 40 milliseconds of the T wave. Unlike first transit studies, which collect the data while the entire radioactive bolus is in the heart, only a fraction of the injected tracer is in the central blood pool under equilibrium conditions. There are insufficient counts in any single 40 or 60-millisecond interval from one cardiac cycle to yield a high quality image. Therefore, data are collected and integrated from several hundred heart cycles until adequate counting statistics are compiled.[4] A sample case is provided in

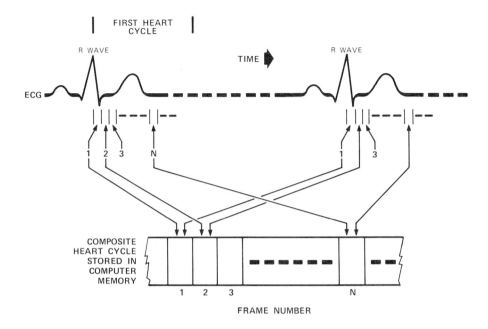

Figure 13-1. Gating concept. In dual gated studies only the end diastolic and end systolic frames are collected. In multigated studies, sequential frames of equal duration are obtained throughout the cardiac cycle.

Figure 13-2 to illustrate the need for gating and building up composite images.

In the original technique, the gating device was used to control recording of analog images.[4] The R wave of the ECG can also be used to control computer acquisition;[6] and with current computer methods, multiframe acquisition formats have been developed which provide a series of images spanning the entire cardiac cycle, much as the multiple images in a contrast cine-ventriculogram represent this cycle.[10,31,32] The acronym "MUGA" (multiple gated acquisition) is now often used to refer to radionuclide ventriculograms obtained in the multi-frame format (Fig. 13-1). Figure 13-3 is a schematic diagram illustrating the direct input of both scintillation data and the gating signals to a computer which becomes the master controller for the entire study.

The duration of an individual frame in multi-frame studies is varied depending on the heart rate to insure adequate temporal resolution.[33] Typical duration for each frame is approximately 30 to 50 milliseconds. In multi-frame studies, the need for identifying end systole electronically is eliminated. End systole is readily identified in the same way it is

SAMPLE ACQUISITION PARAMETERS FOR GATED BLOOD POOL IMAGING

1. Total count rate in gamma camera field of view — 15,000 Counts/Sec

2. Width of gating interval
   (Frame duration)   — 40 Milliseconds

3. Heart rate   — 72 Beats/Minute

4. Total counts required per image   — 300,000 Counts

5. Calculate length of time required for imaging

$$\frac{1 \ \text{Gating Interval}}{\text{Heart Cycle}} \ x \ \frac{40 \ \text{Milliseconds}}{\frac{\text{Gating Interval}}{1000 \ \text{Milliseconds}}} \ x \ \frac{15,000 \ \text{Counts}}{\text{Second}} = \frac{600 \ \text{Counts}}{\text{Heart Cycle}}$$

$$\frac{300,000 \ \text{Counts}}{\frac{600 \ \text{Counts}}{\text{Heart Cycle}}} \ x \ \frac{60 \ \text{Seconds}}{\frac{72}{\text{Heart Cycle}}} = 425 \ \text{Seconds}$$

Figure 13-2.   Sample acquisition parameters. Once the count rate in the gamma camera field-of-view and the patient's heart rate are known, the length of time required for imaging can be calculated based on the desired window width and the desired number of counts per image. The wider the window width or, in the case of multi-frame studies, the longer the duration of each individual frame, the shorter the length of imaging time required for a given number of counts. Note that the calculated imaging time is for the entire study and not just one view since the data are acquired for all images synchronously.

identified in contrast ventriculography, by the frame in which the ventricle appears smallest.

A fundamental assumption underlying the gated or R wave synchronized approach to data collection in radionuclide ventriculography is that the heart cycle remain essentially unchanged throughout the time of data collection. Slight fluctuations in heart rate are inevitable with respiration but significant changes in R-R interval cause time volume relationships in the cardiac cycle to change, thereby invalidating the gating assumption. Premature ventricular contractions (PVC's) or atrial fibrillation with irregular ventricular response cause an unacceptable variation of heart cycles. Therefore the heart rhythm must be documented (Fig. 13-3).

Most laboratories have found it advantageous to take views in several

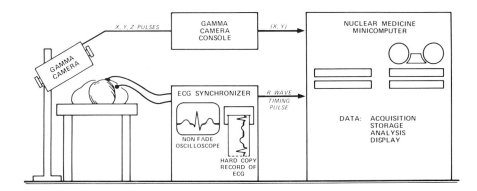

Figure 13-3. Schematic diagram illustrating the concept of computer controlled data acquisition in gated blood pool imaging. The computer also is used to store, analyze and display the data.

projections. It is feasible to take a series of images since the tracers remain in the vascular space over many hours. The single most important view in gated blood pool imaging is the left anterior oblique view (LAO) because the left ventricular blood pool can be distinguished from radioactivity in other cardiac structures. Proper sampling from the left ventricle is necessary for accurate quantitative analysis of left ventricular function. The exact angulation between patient and camera which best isolates the left ventricular blood pool is determined empirically in each case and may vary from 20° to 60°. In practice the gamma camera head is placed in a nominal 40° LAO and the angle systematically varied until the interventricular septum is optimally visualized. At 15° to 20° caudal tilt aids separation of the left ventricle from the left atrium in some patients.

To date, most centers performing equilibrium blood pool imaging have used single crystal gamma scintillation cameras as the imaging device. There are no absolute reasons that the studies could not also be performed on multi-crystal cameras. However, target-to-background ratios are much lower at equilibrium than during first transit. The superior spatial and energy resolution of single crystal gamma cameras are a decided advantage in accurately detecting and outlining ventricular borders in equilibrium images.

Choice of collimation for the gamma camera depends in part on the application. For example, in intervention studies during exercise stress or following administration of a drug, high sensitivity collimators offer significant advantages in reducing data collection intervals. Short collection intervals are necessary to "capture" the functional changes resulting from the intervention. Transient changes in ventricular performance may be lost by data averaging if data collection periods are too long. For studies with the patient at rest, the data collection time is less critical and a low energy, parallel hole, all purpose or even high resolution collimator may be used.

As with first transit studies, probes have also been adapted for blood pool studies.[34,35] Their major advantages and disadavantages are similar to those described for transit procedures.

Advantages and Disadvantages of First Pass Versus Equilibrium Blood Pool Techniques

Universal agreement has not been reached on which of the major data acquisition techniques is superior and the topic has promoted spirited scientific and commercial debate. In the final analysis, the particular requirements of a given laboratory may be more important in deciding which technique to adopt than any theoretical arguments. The major advantages of the first pass technique are the short time required to collect data and the freedom to choose patient position. With appropriate timing, right ventricular function may be analyzed as well as left ventricular function. Short data collection intervals have a theoretical advantage for intervention studies where ventricular function is constantly changing and prolonged sampling is therefore not desirable.

The major disadvantage of the first pass technique is the necessity of administering additional radioactivity for each study and each additional view.[16] This limits the number of sequential studies that may be taken following response to therapy or during an intervention (e.g., drug therapy, exercise stress) and limits the number of views that can be taken to analyze regional wall motion. If new short-lived radionuclides are developed, this disadvantage would be eliminated. Another practical problem in first pass studies is the length of time required to analyze data. A large number of data frames and or scintillation events are recorded and depending on the specifications of the computer system being used. As much as 15 to 45 minutes is required to calculate the quantitative function parameters. Some laboratories with heavy demands on instrumentation have had to defer data analysis until after clinic hours because of this problem. Delay between study performance and results reporting diminishes the clinical impact of the information.

The greatest single advantage of equilibrium blood pool imaging is that multiple views may be taken and studies may be repeated over a prolonged period of time after only a single injection of radiotracer.

Repeat studies allow serial analysis of ventricular function during progressive exercise, in response to drug or other intervention procedures, and during acute episodes such as cardiogenic shock or following cardiac arrest. Data processing times for calculating quantitative function parameters are shorter with equilibrium blood pool imaging because of the gating technique. With gating or synchronizing of data collection, data formatting is done in real time during data acquisition and, in general, no more than five minutes of computer time is required following the completion of a study to calculate the ejection fraction and other quantitative parameters.

A major disadvantage of the gated blood pool technique is the necessity to image over a relatively long period of time. In the original dual gated technique, 10 to 15 minutes were required per view.[4] With currently available programs, however, the time has been reduced to one to two minutes without sacrificing quantitative accuracy. Nonetheless, imaging time is a limitation which must be considered, particularly for radionuclide ventriculography during exercise (see below). A second disadvantage of the gated blood pool technique is that the left ventricle cannot be completely isolated from other structures in all views. For example, in the right anterior oblique view, activity in the right ventricle usually superimposes the inferior wall and part of the septum and base of the left ventricle. A corollary to this observation is that unmodified gated blood pool studies cannot be used to analyze right ventricular function quantitatively.

In current practice, the equilibrium blood pool approach to radionuclide ventriculography and analysis of left ventricular function is being used in a larger number of centers than is the first pass technique, primarily because most nuclear medicine clinics have single crystal gamma scintillation cameras as standard imaging devices. In addition, the cost of adding a small dedicated minicomputer to control the acquisition of data and analyze and display quantitative data (Fig. 13-3) is substantially less than the cost of a separate multi-crystal camera with computer for first transit studies. Also, using mobile cameras to do radionuclide ventriculography in areas remote from the nuclear imaging clinic has become an important new application. To date, only single crystal camera systems are available for mobile applications and again, the greater suitability of this type of instrument for equilibrium blood pool imaging rather than first pass imaging has favored use of the former technique.

Data Analysis—Information Available

Complete analysis of radionuclide ventriculograms includes both qualitative and quantitative observations. Qualitative information is derived by direct inspection of the nuclear images and includes estimates of ventricular size and configuration and detection of abnormalities in regional wall motion. Quantitative information is derived from numerical data processing. The most important calculated parameter is the ejection fraction. Estimates of ventricular emptying rates and other quantitative parameters are also available depending on the format used to collect data.

Detection of Abnormalities in Regional Wall Motion

Zaret and co-workers first described the use of nuclear gated blood pool imaging to detect abnormalities in regional wall motion in 1971.[36] In their approach, the left ventricular contour was outlined by hand tracing from gated analog images taken at end diastole and end systole. The edge outlines were then superimposed on each other providing a method for assessing wall excursion between end diastole and end systole. Less than 20 percent shortening of the hemiaxis of the left ventricle was considered indicative of ventricular wall hypokinesis.[36] At points of ventricular wall akinesis, the traced outlines exactly superimposed and dyskinesis was readily identified where the end systolic outline projected beyond the limits of the end diastolic outline. This general approach remains a valid one and has been adapted by other investigators for detecting wall motion abnormalities from computer-generated ventricular outlines.[13,16,18,19] Figure 13-4 illustrates this technique. Figures 13-4A and 13-4B are the end diastolic and end systolic computer-generated left ventricular outlines, respectively. In Figure 13-4C the outlines are added together. The edges superimpose along the posterolateral margin indicating an akinetic wall segment.

Abnormal wall motion may also be detected by using the nuclear medicine computer to replay the data in cinematic display format. An endless loop is created and displayed continuously on the computer oscilloscope or videoscreen. The contraction of the left ventricle may be followed repeatedly throughout a multiple frame radionuclide ventriculogram. Systematic inspection of the ventricular wall segments is done in a manner analogous to inspection of contrast ventriculograms.

Yet another method for detecting regional wall motion abnormalities is the "difference" image or "stroke volume" image formed by subtracting the end systolic frame point by point from the end diastolic

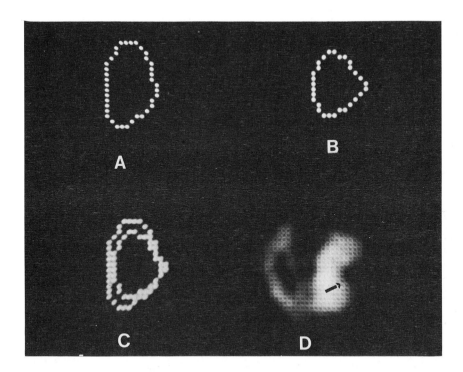

Figure 13-4.   *A* and *B* are computer generated edges of the left ventricle at end diastole and end systole respectively. In *C* the computer has been used to add the edge outlines together. The patient was imaged in the left anterior oblique position. The edge outlines superimpose laterally indicating akinesis in the distribution of the circumflex artery. The difference image or stroke volume image is presented in *D*. There is a clear cut defect (arrow) in the portion of the image adjacent to the akinetic wall segment. This was confirmed on the cinematic display as well.

frame[10,13] (Figs. 13-4*D* and 13-5). In this type of functional image, regions of high stroke volume are depicted as intense areas. In regions where little or no blood has been expelled, the display is less intense or blank. By displaying the stroke volume image along with a superimposed end diastolic outline (Fig. 13-5*B*), areas of poor regional function are readily detected and related to ventricular anatomy. Stroke volume images are of particular value when abnormal wall segments are not forming the border in the image. For example, the apex is often projected onto the middle of the left ventricular image in the left anterior oblique view and therefore apical wall motion abnormalities may escape detection in the cinematic display or by analysis of edge outlines. In such cases the stroke volume image is of particular value. Studies using all

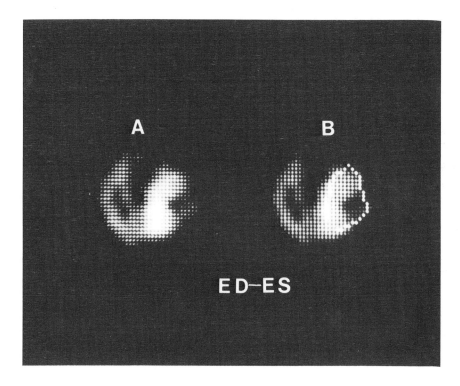

Figure 13-5. *A*, The stroke volume image from the same patient as in Figure 13-4 with the end diastolic edge superimposed in *B*. Superimposing the edge is simply a way of better documenting the location of the defect.

these approaches have shown favorable correlations between nuclear and contrast ventriculographic detection of abnormalities in regional wall motion abnormalities.[12,13,16,18,19]

Quantitative Analysis

Computational methods for determining the ejection fraction depend on the mode of data acquisition. For equilibrium gated blood pool imaging, the ejection fraction may be calculated using either an adaptation of contrast angiographic "area-length" formulae as originally described by Strauss[4] or by using the "time-activity" method first proposed by Parker.[6] If only analog images are available, the area length method must be used. Currently, in centers where computers are available, the time-activity method is preferred. The rationale underlying this method is that the amount of radioactivity in the ventricle is proportional to blood volume in each ventricle at each point in the cardiac cycle. The left ventricle and the area just outside the ventricle (to correct for background activity) are flagged on the computer as regions of interest. The ejection fraction is calculated from the net count at end diastole and the net count at end systole. Figure 13-6 represents a sample calculation including the steps necessary to correct for background radioactivity.

Recently, semi-automatic edge programs have been developed to help delineate the left ventricular contour and automatically flag computer regions of interest.[37] Such programs reduce variation among observers in the numerical calculation of ejection fraction and also facilitate frame by frame analysis throughout the cardiac cycle. Using a semi-automatic edge detection program, Burow and co-workers demonstrated good correlation between both the radionuclide ejection fraction and the frame-by-frame ventricular volumes calculated by both radionuclide and contrast ventriculography.[37] Figure 13-7 illustrates the steps in processing

EJECTION FRACTION: SAMPLE CALCULATION

I. Formula:

$$\text{Ejection Fraction} = \frac{\text{End Diastolic Counts (Net)} - \text{End Systolic Counts (Net)}}{\text{End Diastolic Counts (Net)}}$$

II. Sample Data:

	End Diastole	End Systole
Number of Channels in Left Ventricular Region of Interest	118	89
Counts per Channel	119	106
Background Counts per Channel	48	48

III. Calculations

Net End Diastolic Counts   = (118 x 119) — (118 x 48)

                           = 8353

Net End Systolic Counts   = (106 x 89) — (106 x 48)

                           = 5190

Ejection Fraction   = $\dfrac{8353 - 5190}{8353}$

                           = .38

Figure 13-6. Sample ejection fraction calculation. The numbers are taken from an actual case. Separate end-diastolic and end-systolic regions of interest were flagged for the left ventricle using a computer light pen. Regions of interest may also be defined by semi-automatic edge detection algorithms with the aid of computers.

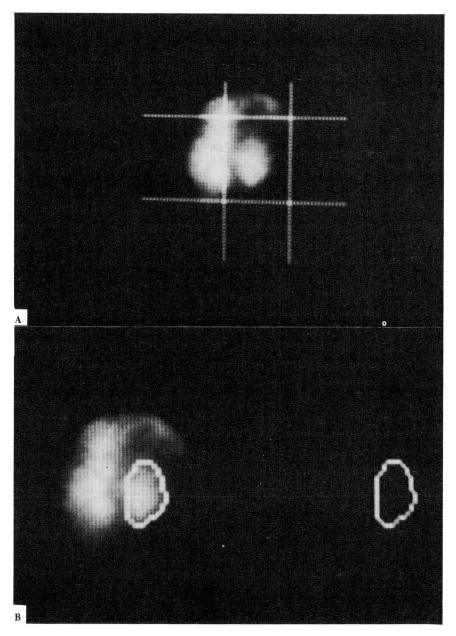

Figure 13-7. Steps in automated data processing. In *A* the computer operator has defined an "expectation" window using cursors to tell the computer program the approximate region of the left ventricle. Part *B* illustrates the computer detected end-diastolic outline with and without the outline superimposed on the end-diastolic image. By direct visual inspection the outline corresponds well with the borders of the left ventricle. The computer operator inspects each frame to insure that the algorithm has not failed.

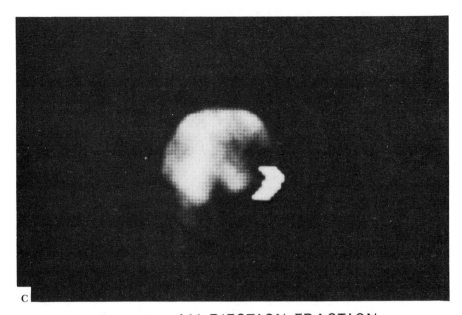

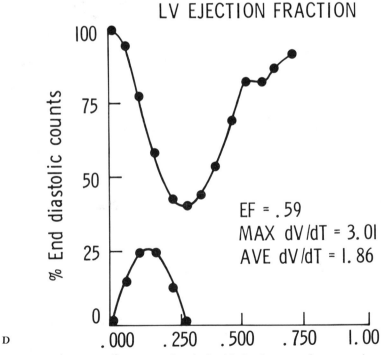

Figure 13-7 (Continued).   In panel *C* the highlighted region adjacent to the ventricle is the computer selected background area obtained in the end systolic frame. The time activity curve and the numerical calculations of ejection fraction and fractional ejection rate are presented in *D*. The lower curve is simply the first derivative of the upper curve and is a measure of the fractional ejection rate between each two frames of the gated blood pool study.

the computer data and the computer-generated time-activity curve from multi-frame radionuclide ventriculogram.

Methods for quantitative analysis in first transit studies are generally similar to those described above. Background corrected time-activity curves are generated; net ventricular counts are determined at end diastole and end systole; and the ejection fraction, calculated with the same formula described for equilibrium blood pool imaging. Fig. 13-8 illustrates regions of interest flagged for the left ventricle and background in a first transit study. Figure 13-9 depicts the background corrected left ventricular time-activity curve. The best numerical correlations between first pass radionuclide and contrast angiographic ejection fractions are made from data collected immediately following peak activity in the left ventricle[11] (Fig.13-9). Since the location of these data frames is not known before the data are analyzed, they must be iden-

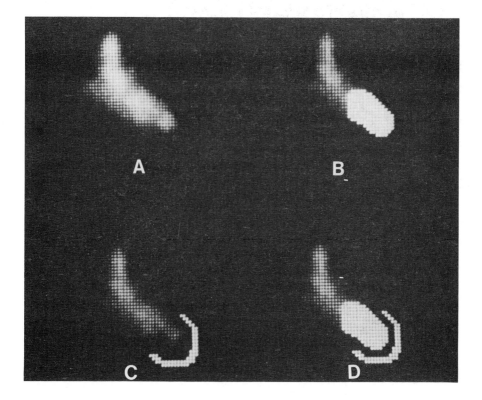

Figure 13-8.   Panel *A* illustrates a composite end-diastolic frame from a first transit radionuclide ventriculogram. *B* and *C* illustrate the left ventricular and background regions of interest respectively. They are both superimposed on the image in *D*.

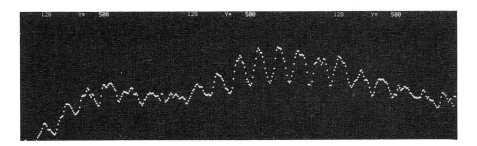

Figure 13-9.   Time activity curve from the study illustrated in Figure 13-8. The curve was generated from the left ventricular region of interest. The cyclical fluctuations and low peak early in the curve are due to activity in the right ventricle which partially superimposes the left ventricle. There is then a relatively flat portion of the curve while the activity is predominantly in the lungs followed by rapid increase in activity during the left ventricular phase. Ejection fraction may be calculated either beat by beat or data from sequential heart cycles during the peak left ventricular activity may be added together for greater statistical reliability.

tified by generating a time-activity curve from a provisional region of interest marked in the left ventricle. A second, more accurate left ventricular region of interest is then flagged from a summed image of selected data frames immediately following peak left ventricular activity and a true left ventricular time-activity curve generated.[11,13,18] The ejection fraction may be calculated on a beat-to-beat basis by taking end diastole from local peaks on the curve and end systole from the following valleys. To improve statistical reliability, the ejection fraction is usually averaged for several beats.[11,13,18]

Calculation of regional ejection fractions as well as the global ejection fraction has also recently been described.[38] This may be done (1) pixel by pixel, by dividing the stroke volume image described above by the end diastolic image which has been corrected for background radiation or (2) by dividing the end systolic image into multiple pie-shaped segments and calculating the ejection fraction of each segment. In the ejection fraction image, areas of good function are portrayed by high intensity of radioactivity while areas bordered by hypokinetic or akinetic wall segments demonstrate low image intensities.

Numerous centers have now made correlations of nuclear ejection fractions by a variety of data collection and analysis techniques and compared then to the ejection fraction values obtained from contrast ventriculography.[4,8,9,12,19,37,39,40] Table 13-1 summarizes some of the results: the data collection technique, the method of calculation and the number of subjects studied are indicated as well as the correlation

TABLE 13-1

Correlation of Ejection Fractions Calculated By Radionuclide and Contrast Ventriculography

Author Reference No.	Radionuclide Technique	Method of Calculation	Number of Patients	Correlation Coefficient (r)
Strauss[4]	Equilibrium ECG gated ED°, ES°°	Geometric Area-Length	20	.92
Berman[12]	Equilibrium ECG and phono gated ED, ES	Area-Length	27	.93
Secker-Walker[8]	Equilibrium ECG gated ED, ES	Time-Activity	10	.87
Ashburn[9]	First Pass	Area-Length	13	.94
Schelbert[11]	First Pass	Time-Activity	20	.94
Pavel[19]	First Pass	Time-Activity	40	.89
Burrow[37]	Equilibrium Multiple Gated	Time-Activity	17	.93
Folland[39]	a,b) Equilibrium Multiple Gated	a) Time-Activity	30	.84
		b) Area-Length	30	.73
	c) First Pass	c) Time-Activity	30	.86
Green[40]	Equilibrium Multiple Gated	Time-Activity	39	.92

° ED: End-diastole
°° ES: End-systole

coefficient. One can conclude from these uniformly good results derived from experience in a variety of centers that calculation of the ejection fraction by radionuclide left ventriculography is highly accurate.

Although contrast ventriculography remains the standard for comparison, there are theoretical reasons to suggest the potential superiority of the radionuclide method in some settings. For unusual ventricular shapes and in conditions where significant regional abnormalities exist in ventricular wall motion, the radionuclide approach may well be more accurate. For instance, in patients with ventricular aneurysms, and in patients with ventricular enlargement, the assumption that the ventricle can be approximated by an ellipsoid of revolution is not correct. In radionuclide ventriculography with time-activity analysis, no geometric assumptions are necessary.

References

1. Dodge, H.T., Sandler, H., Baxley, W.A., et al.: Usefulness and limitations of radiographic methods for determining left ventricular volume. *Am J Cardiol* **18**:10-24, 1966
2. Prinzmetal, M., Corday, E., Spritzler, R.J., et al.: Radiocardiography and its clinical applications. *JAMA* **139**:617-622, 1949.
3. Mullins, C.B., Mason, D.T., Ashburn, W.L., et al.: Determination of ventricular volume by radioisotope-angiography. *Am J Cardiol* **24**:72-78, 1969.
4. Strauss, H.W., Zaret, B.L., Hurley, P.J., et al.: A scintiphotographic method for measuring left ventricular ejection fraction in man without cardiac catheterization. *Am J Cardiol* **28**:575-580, 1971.
5. Van Dyke, D., Anger, H.O., Sullivan, R.W., et al.: Cardiac evaluation from radioisotope dynamics. *J Nucl Med* **13**:585-592, 1972.
6. Parker, J.A., Secker-Walker, R., Hill, R., et al.: A new technique for the calculation of left ventricular ejection fraction. *J Nucl Med* **13**:649-651, 1972.
7. Weber, P.M., dos Remedios, L.V., and Jasko, I.A.: Quantitative radioisotopic angiocardiography. *J Nucl Med* **13**:815-822, 1972.
8. Secker-Walker, R.H., Resnick, L., Kunz, H., et al.: Measurement of left ventricular ejection fraction. *J Nucl Med* **14**:798-802, 1973.
9. Ashburn, W.L., Kostuk, W.J., Karliner, J.S., et al.: Left ventricular volume and ejection fraction determination by radionuclide angiography. *Sem Nucl Med* **3**:165-176, 1973.
10. Green, M.V., Ostrow, H.G., Douglas, M.A., et al.: High temporal resolution ECG-gated scintigraphic angiocardiography. *J Nucl Med* **16**:95-98, 1975.
11. Schelbert, H.R., Verba, J.W., Johnson, A.D., et al.: Nontraumatic determination of left ventricular ejection fraction by radionuclide angiocardiography. *Circulation* **51**:902-909, 1975.

12. Berman, D.S., Salel, A.F., DeNardo, G.L., et al.: Clinical assessment of left ventricular regional contraction patterns and ejection fraction by high-resolution gated scintigraphy. *J Nucl Med* **16**:865-874, 1975.

13. Schad, N.: Nontraumatic assessment of left ventricular wall motion and regional stroke volume after myocardial infarction. *J Nucl Med* **18**:333-341, 1977.

14. Watson, D.D., Nelson, J.P., and Gottlieb, S.: Rapid bolus injection of radioisotopes. *Radiology* **106**:347-352, 1973.

15. Bowyer, K.W., Konstantinow, G., Rerych, S.K., et al.: Optimum counting intervals in radionuclide cardiac studies. In *Nuclear Cardiology: Selected Computer Aspects*, Symposium Proceedings, Society of Nuclear Medicine, Atlanta, Georgia, 1978, pp. 85-95.

16. Berger, H.J., Gottschalk, A., Zaret, B.L.: First-pass radionuclide angiocardiography for evaluation of right and left ventricular performance: computer applications and technical considerations. In *Nuclear Cardiology: Selected Computer Aspects*, Symposium Proceedings, Society of Nuclear Medicine, Atlanta, Georgia, 1978, pp. 29-44.

17. Murphy, P., Arseneau, R., Maxon, E., et al.: Clinical significance of scintillation camera electronics capable of high processing gates. *J Nucl Med* **18**:175-179, 1977.

18. Hecht, H.S., Mirell, S.G., Rolett, E.L., et al.: Left-ventricular ejection fraction and segmental wall motion by peripheral first-pass radionuclide angiography. *J Nucl Med* **19**:17-23, 1978.

19. Pavel, D.G., Byron, E., Ayers, B., et al.: Multifaceted evaluation of left ventricular function by the first transit technique using Anger-type cameras and an optimized protocol: Correlation with biplane roentgen angiography. In *Nuclear Cardiology: Selected Computer Aspects*, Symposium Proceedings, Society of Nuclear Medicine, Atlanta, Georgia, 1978, pp. 129-138.

20. Steele, P.P., Van Dyke, D., Trow, R.S., et al.: Simple and safe bedside method for serial measurement of left ventricular ejection fraction, cardiac output and pulmonary blood volume. *Br Heart J* **36**:122-131, 1974.

21. Berndt, T., Alderman, E.L., Wasnich, R., et al.: Evaluation of portable radionuclide method for measurement of left ventricular ejection fraction and cardiac output. *J Nucl Med* **16**:289-292, 1975.

22. Groch, M.W., Gottlieb, S., Mallon, S.M., et al.: A new dual-probe system for the rapid bedside assessment of left ventricular function. *J Nucl Med* **17**:930-936, 1976.

23. Eckelman, W., Richards, P., Hauser, W., et al.: Technetium-labeled red blood cells. *J Nucl Med* **12**:22-24, 1971.

24. Bardy, A., Fouyé, H., Gobin, R., et al.: Technetium-99m labeling by means of stannous pyrophosphate: Application to bleomycin and red blood cells. *J Nucl Med* **16**:435-437, 1975.

25. Smith, T.D., and Richards, P.: A simple kit for preparation of ^{99m}Tc-labeled red blood cells. *J Nucl Med* **17**:126-132, 1976.

26. Pavel, D.G., Zimmer, A.M., and Patterson, V.N.: In vivo labeling of red blood cells with ^{99m}Tc: A new approach to blood pool visualization. *J Nucl Med* **18**:305-308, 1977.

27. Hamilton, R.G., and Alderson, P.O.: A comparative evaluation of techniques for rapid and efficient in vivo labeling of red cells with (^{99m}Tc) pertechnetate. *J Nucl Med* **18**:1010-1013, 1977.

28. Stokely, E.M., Parkey, R.W., Bonte, F.J., et al.: Gated blood pool imaging following ^{99m}Tc stannous pyrophosphate imaging. *Radiology* **120**:433-434, 1976.

29. Heege, F.N., Hamilton, G.W., Larson, S.M., et al.: Cardiac chamber imaging: A comparison of red blood cells labeled with Tc-99m in vitro and in vivo. *J Nucl Med* **19**:129-134, 1978.

30. Thrall, J.H., Freitas, J.E., Swanson, D.P., et al.: Clinical comparison of cardiac blood pool visualization with technetium-99m red blood cells labeled in vivo and with technetium human serum albumin. *J Nucl Med* **19**:796-803, 1978.

31. Strauss, H.W., Singleton, R., Burow, R., et al.: Multiple gated acquisition (MUGA): An improved noninvasive technique for evaluation of regional wall motion (RWM) and left ventricular function (LVF). *Am J Cardiol* **39**:284, 1977 (Abstract).

32. Bacharach, S.L., Greene, M.V., Borer, J.S., et al.: A real-time system for multi-image gated cardiac studies. *J Nucl Med* **18**: 79-84, 1977.

33. Hamilton, G.W., Williams, D.L., and Caldwell, J.H.: Frame-rate requirements for recording time-activity curves by radionuclide angiography. In *Nuclear Cardiology: Selected Computer Aspects*, Symposium Proceedings, Society of Nuclear Medicine, Atlanta, Georgia, 1978, pp. 85-96.

34. Wagner, H.N., Wake, R., Nickoloff, E., et al.: The nuclear stethoscope: A simple device for generation of left ventricular volume curves. *Am J Cardiol* **38**:747-750, 1976.

35. Bacharach, S.L., Greene, M.V., Borer, J.S., et al.: ECG-gated scintillation probe measurement of left ventricular function. *J Nucl Med* **18**:1176-1183, 1977.

36. Zaret, B.L., Strauss, H.W., Hurley, P.J., et al.: A noninvasive scintiphotographic method for detecting regional ventricular dysfunction in man. *N Engl J Med* **284**:1165-1170, 1971.

37. Burow, R.D., Strauss, H.W., Singleton, R., et al.: Analysis of left ventricular function from multiple gated acquisition cardiac blood pool imaging. Comparison to contrast angiography. *Circulation* **56**:1024-1028, 1977.

38. Maddox, D.E., Holman, B.L., Wynne, J., et al.: Ejection fraction image: A non-invasive index of regional left ventricular wall motion. *Am J Cardiol* **41**:1230-1238, 1978.

39. Folland, E.D., Hamilton, G.W., Larson, S.M., et al.: The radionuclide ejection fraction: A comparison of three radionuclide techniques with contrast angiography. *J Nucl Med* **18**:1159-1166, 1977.

40. Greene, M.V., Brody, W.R., Douglas, M.A., et al.: Ejection fraction by count rate from gated images. *J Nucl Med* **19**:880-883, 1978.

CHAPTER XIV

Clinical Applications of Radionuclide Ventriculography

James H. Thrall, M.D.
Bertram Pitt, M.D.
Thomas J. Brady, M.D.

Radionuclide ventriculography has now been used to study a wide spectrum of cardiac disorders requiring assessment of global and regional left ventricular function.[1-5,9] This procedure was first used to evaluate patients who had myocardial infarctions and those with left ventricular failure. Abnormalities in wall motion and diminished ejection fractions can be detected in a large percentage of patients who have had recent acute myocardial infarctions.[5,6] Prognosis for patients leaving the hospital after having acute infarcts has been shown to be much worse for patients with low ejection fractions than for those with normal or only slightly compromised left ventricular function. In patients with congestive heart failure, the radionuclide study has been helpful in detecting left ventricular aneurysms as the cause of failure and in distinguishing this condition from diffusely poor ventricular function. [7,8]

These two clinical applications are discussed in detail elsewhere in this text. A more recent application of radionuclide ventriculography is in evaluating patients with stable coronary artery disease where ventricular function is often normal under resting conditions. Borer and co-workers introduced the technique of radionuclide ventriculography during exercise for evaluating such patients. The rationale for the exercise phase of the ventriculogram is essentially identical to that for the exercise treadmill test. Coronary blood flow and myocardial perfusion are adequate at rest but during exercise stress, imbalances between oxygen supply and demand develop and ventricular dysfunction can be detected. Although stress radionuclide ventriculography is a relatively new procedure, exercise protocols have already been developed for both gamma cameras and scintillation probes with either first pass or equilibrium gated blood pool methods of data acquisition.[10]

In his original studies Borer used the equilibrium gated blood pool approach. With this technique left anterior oblique views are taken with the patient lying supine. A baseline study documents resting ventricular function. The patient then begins pedalling a bicycle equipped with ergometer, and a second study is done during maximal exercise. Even with new computer routines, the data acquisition requires 60 to 120 seconds of imaging time, an important practical point. The termination of exercise must be anticipated to allow sufficient data acquisition time at conditions of maximal achievable stress. The relatively short time required for data acquisition with the first pass technique is an advantage for stress radionuclide ventriculography. However, this technique requires two injections of the radiotracer.[3]

From a technical standpoint, there are more disadvantages to doing radionuclide ventriculography with the patient exercising than with the patient at rest. The disadvantages include the need to acquire and integrate the function of accessory equipment such as the bicycle ergometer; the need to develop an exercise protocol and the skills for monitoring patients during exercise stress; and the increased need to train personnel for responding to emergencies.

Normal subjects and patients without significant coronary artery disease increase their ejection fractions with exercise from a resting mean of approximately 60 to 65 percent to an exercise mean 10 to 20 percent higher. Figure 14-1 illustrates the time-activity curves and ejection fraction calculations at rest and during exercise in a patient later shown to have normal coronary arteries. The ejection fraction during maximal exercise increased 17 percentage points compared to the resting value. Figure 14-2 illustrates the respective end diastolic and end systolic frames from the resting and exercise studies. The end-diastolic ventricular volumes are essentially identical. During exercise the end-systolic volume is clearly smaller, accounting for the higher ejection fraction.

Patients with ischemic heart disease show either a decrease in the ejection fraction or a failure to increase the ejection fraction beyond the statistical variability of the determination. The time-activity curves for a patient with a high grade left anterior descending artery stenosis were calculated with the patient at rest and exercising (Fig. 14-3). The corresponding end-diastolic and end-systolic images are illustrated in Figure 14-4. The end-diastolic volume has increased only slightly while the end-systolic volume during exercise is significantly increased, accounting for most of the decline in the ejection fraction. Figure 14-5 illustrates the functional stroke volume images taken at rest and during exercise. A

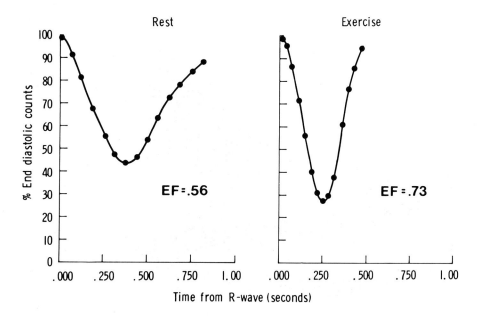

Figure 14-1. Panels *A* and *B* illustrate the time activity curves obtained at rest and during maximal exercise, respectively, in a patient subsequently shown not to have coronary artery disease. The frame duration reflects the actual heart rates at which the two studies were obtained. Note that the ejection fraction increases significantly during exercise.

distinct defect along the inferior border of the apex and the septum indicates the involvement of the left anterior descending artery by indicating the site of regional dysfunction. Patients with chest pain of noncardiac origin show a normal increase in ejection fraction during exercise. The fact is of major clinical importance since the differentiation of patients with atypical chest pain is necessary to avoid unnecessary coronary arteriography with its associated risks and expense.

Although clinical experience is still limited, the reported sensitivity for detection of ischemic heart disease by exercise radionuclide ventriculography is over 90 percent.[10-12] The degree of sensitivity has not been uniformly duplicated in all centers.[3] Undoubtedly there will be an irreducible percentage of false negative examination as there is with any diagnostic procedure, but sufficient experience has been reported to indicate that the sensitivity is adversely affected by inadequate technique. In addition to inaccurate data analysis, the major pitfall is the patient's failure to achieve maximal exercise levels. The need for ade-

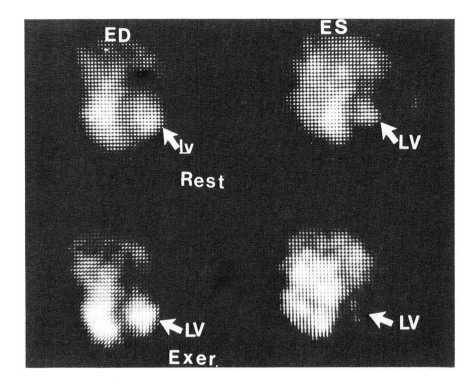

Figure 14-2. Selected end-diastolic and end-systolic frames during rest and exercise from the same patient as Figure 14-1. Note the much smaller end-systolic volume of the left ventricle during exercise with the relative lack of change in the end-diastolic appearance.

quate exercise during testing of some patients is perhaps best illustrated by the results of graded exercise imaging (Fig. 14-6 to 14-8). Normal individuals usually increase their ejection fractions to a plateau value in the range of 75 to 85 percent. Patients with ischemic heart disease demonstrate a number of response patterns. In some, the left ventricular ejection fraction declines even at the lowest exercise level and falls progressively. In these patients function deteriorates as exercise causes increased ischemia (Fig. 14-7). In other patients, however, the left ventricular ejection fraction may increase initially. It falls only at high exercise levels and may remain significantly above the baseline value (Fig. 14-8). In a pilot series reported by Berger and co-workers, studies were done with the patient both resting and exercising vigorously. In nine of thirteen patients with angiographically proven coronary artery disease, exercise was limited by leg fatigue rather than angina, and each of the nine patients had a rise in ejection fraction.[3] Experience at the

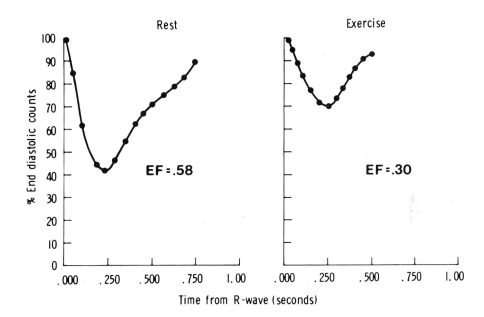

LEFT VENTRICULAR TIME - ACTIVITY CURVES

Figure 14-3.   Time activity curves at rest and exercise in a patient with a 99 percent stenosis of the left anterior descending artery. Resting function is within normal limits. During exercise the ejection fraction falls essentially in half.

University of Michigan Medical Center has been similar. Coronary artery disease was detected by radionuclide ventriculography in 56 of 57 patients who exercised adequately. Adequate exercise is defined as exercise causing chest pain or a pressure-rate-product greater than 250 (heart rate x systolic blood pressure/100). On the other hand, four of thirteen patients with coronary artery disease were unable to exercise sufficiently because of leg fatigue. These four patients had false negative examinations and the increase in ejection fraction averaged an absolute 12 percent. These results indicate that when exercise levels are inadequate, either because of poor technique, fatigue, or inability to exercise, the recording of an increase in ejection fraction is increased and sensitivity for detecting coronary disease is reduced.

In addition to the ejection fraction response, a high percentage of patients with coronary artery disease develop regional abnormalities in wall motion with exercise. These abnormalities are readily appreciated on the dynamic cinematic display as areas of decreased motion. If ischemic segments do not form borders in the image, functional images

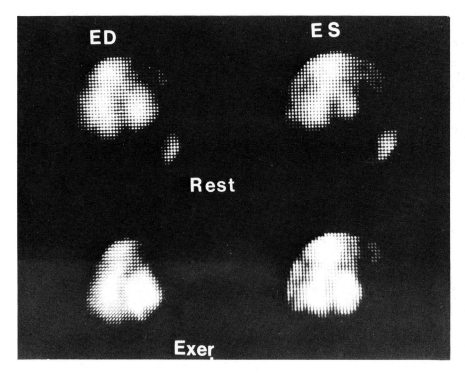

Figure 14-4. End diastolic and end systolic frames during rest and exercise from the same patient as Figure 14-3. Note that the end-diastolic volume increases slightly during exercise but the end-systolic volume is markedly enlarged accounting for the substantial decline in ejection fraction.

depicting regional ejection fraction or regional stroke volumes are necessary to appreciate the regional dysfunction[10] (Fig. 14-5).

Radionuclide ventriculography during exercise has also been used to evaluate a number of clinical problems other than the diagnosis of coronary artery disease. The procedure is also useful in evaluating patients for cardiac rehabilitation programs. Patients with marked impairment may be screened out, and those patients judged capable can enter physical training programs. Radionuclide ventriculograms with exercise can be used to evaluate changes in left ventricular performance in patients on physical training programs. With the current national emphasis on cardiac rehabilitation for patients who have had acute myocardial infarctions, this may become a major application.

The effect of therapeutic agents such as vasodilators has also been studied with radionuclide ventriculography by analyzing the response of ejection fraction during exercise.[11] In patients with normal resting

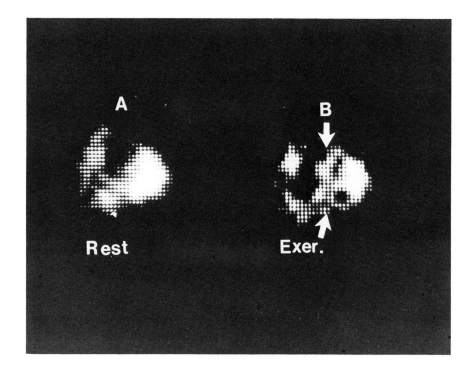

Figure 14-5. Stroke volume or difference images from the same patient as in Figure 14-3 and 14-4. *A*, At rest the stroke volume image is essentially normal. During exercise a mottled area of decreased intensity develops along the septum and inferoapically (arrow); this pinpoints the segmental nature of the ventricular dysfunction developing during exercise.

global and regional function, the efficacy of various drugs can only be assessed by having the patient exercise to a level which would ordinarily induce dysfunction. By comparing radionuclide ventriculograms taken at comparable levels of stress both before and after therapy, the effects of a drug may be assessed objectively.

The same rationale may be used for evaluating patients before and after coronary artery bypass grafting.[12] Before surgery, patients with angina experience a decrease in ejection fractions in response to exercise. A normal exercise response following surgery suggests graft patency and implies relief of ischemia. Continued abnormal exercise response suggests persistence of ischemia. Resting studies showing the development of abnormal wall motion not seen preoperatively or a decrease in the resting ejection fraction suggests perioperative infarction. Following surgery the marked increase in end systolic volume is no longer seen

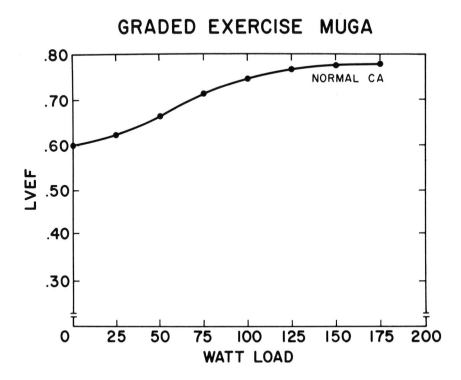

Figure 14-6.   Graded exercise radionuclide ventriculography. In normal subjects the ejection fraction increases with exercise reaching a plateau as the maximum heart rate is approached.

when the patient is exercising (Figs. 14-9 and 14-10).

In valvular heart disease, radionuclide ventriculography during exercise may play a role in planning for surgery. Some patients with asymptomatic aortic regurgitation have an abnormal response to exercise.[13] Such patients may be candidates for valve replacement even though they are asymptomatic. It has been recognized for some time that patients coming to surgery often have irreparable myocardial damage which cannot be corrected by valve replacement. The exercise radionuclide ventriculogram may provide means for detecting functional abnormalities before they are clinically apparent and therefore offering the patient a better chance of recovery.

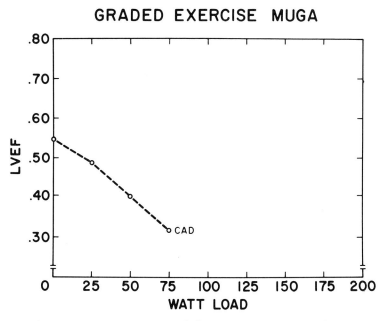

Figure 14-7. Response patterns to graded exercise in patients with coronary artery disease are variable. In the subject illustrated in this figure, the ejection fraction declined at even the lowest exercise levels and ventricular function deteriorated progressively.

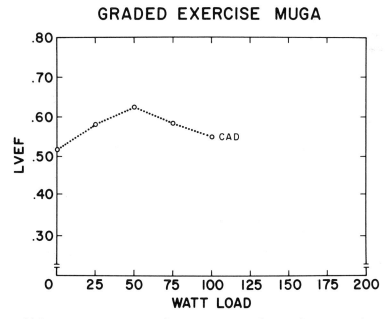

Figure 14-8. In some patients with coronary artery disease the ejection fraction increases at lower levels of exercise. The diagnosis is established in the graded study by the abnormal response at higher levels. If patients with this type of response are only exercised at rest and maximum stress, this study may be interpreted as negative.

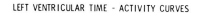

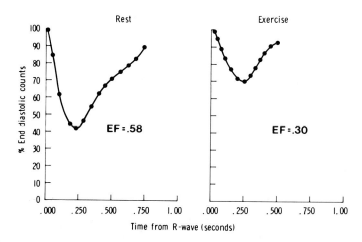

Figure 14-9.   Time activity curves at rest and during exercise following coronary artery bypass in the patient illustrated previously in Figures 14-3, 14-4, and 14-5. Resting function has not changed significantly but the marked decline in ejection fraction with exercise is no longer present. Although the failure to significantly increase the ejection fraction with exercise is not normal, ventricular function is obviously improved.

Conclusions

In less than a decade radionuclide ventriculography has become an accepted and important diagnostic tool. Although current techniques are still being perfected, and newer, more sophisticated procedures are being developed, the basic instrumentation, radiopharmaceuticals and methodology should now be available in any hospital with a department of nuclear medicine. All of the necessary equipment is commercially available from a wide variety of sources.

Future developments will undoubtedly include modifications at every step of most procedures. More sensitive gamma cameras will reduce data collection times. Improvements in automated data analysis will both speed numerical calculations and improve their accuracy. As the value of noninvasive techniques for detecting ventricular dysfunction at the bedside is more widely recognized, further improvements in technology should be forthcoming, especially the development of better mobile scintillation cameras and specialized smaller devices.

In many respects, radionuclide ventriculography is at a crossroads. The techniques have been applied in clinical research studies and validated clinically, but general clinical use is still in its infancy. The development of techniques for detecting ventricular dysfunction during exercise has futher enhanced the utility of the procedure. These techniques and intervention studies of several types may well become the most important applications of radionuclide ventriculography.

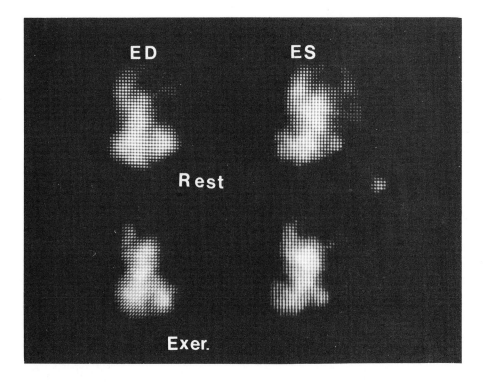

Figure 14-10. Selected end-diastolic and end-systolic frames at rest and during exercise in the same patients as in Figure 14-9 following coronary artery bypass grafting. The end-systolic volume during exercise is much smaller than before the operation. (See Fig. 14-4).

References

1. Berman, D.S., Salel, A.F., DeNardo, G.L., et al.: Clinical assessment of left ventricular regional contraction patterns and ejection fraction by high-resolution gated scintigraphy. *J Nucl Med* **16**: 865-874, 1975.

2. Schad, N.: Nontraumatic assessment of left ventricular wall motion and regional stroke volume after myocardial infarction. *J Nucl Med* **18**: 333-341, 1977.

3. Berger, H.J., Gottschalk, A., and Zaret, B.L.: First-pass radionuclide angiocardiography for evaluation of right and left ventricular performance: computer applications and technical considerations. In *Nuclear Cardiology: Selected Computer Aspects*, Symposium Proceedings, Society of Nuclear Medicine, Atlanta, Georgia, 1978, pp. 29-44.

4. Zaret, B.L., Strauss, H.W., Hurley, P.J., et al.: A noninvasive scintiphotographic method for detecting regional ventricular dysfunction in man. *N Engl J Med* **284**: 1165-1170, 1971.

5. Rigo, P., Murray, M., Strauss, H.W., et al.: Left ventricular function in acute myocardial infarction evaluated by gated scintiphotography. *Circulation* **50**: 678-684, 1974.

6. Rigo, P., Murray, M., Taylor, D.R., et al.: Right ventricular dysfunction detected by gated scintiphotography in patients with acute inferior myocardial infarction. *Circulation* **52**: 268-274, 1975.

7. Rigo, P., Murray, M., Strauss, H.W., et al.: Scintiphotographic evaluation of patients with suspected left ventricular aneurysm. *Circulation* **50**: 985-991, 1974.

8. Schulze, R.A., Strauss, H.W., and Pitt, B.: Sudden death in the year following myocardial infarction: Relation to Ventricular Premature Contractions in the late hospital phase and left ventricular ejection fraction. *Am J Med* **62**: 192-199, 1977.

9. Pitt, B., and Strauss, H.W.: Current concepts: Evaluation of ventricular function by radioisotopic techniques. *N Engl J Med* **296**: 1097-1099, 1977.

10. Borer, J.S., Bacharach, S.L., Green, M.V., et al.: Real-time radionuclide cineangiography in the noninvasive evaluation of global and regional left ventricular function at rest and during exercise in patients with coronary artery disease. *N Engl J Med* **296**: 839-844, 1977.

11. Borer, J.S., Bacharach, S.L., Green, M.V., et al.: Effect of nitroglycerin on exercise-induced abnormalities of left ventricular regional function and ejection fraction in coronary artery disease. Assessment by radionuclide cineangiography in symptomatic and asymptomatic patients. *Circulation* **57**: 314-320, 1978.

12. Kent, K.M., Borer, J.S., and Green, M.V.: Effects of coronary-artery bypass on global and regional left ventricular function during exercise. *N Engl J Med* **298**: 1434-1439, 1978.

13. Borer, J.S., Bacharach, S.L., and Green, M.V.: Left ventricular function during exercise before and after aortic valve replacement. *Circulation* **55** and **56**: III-28, 1977 (Abstract).

CHAPTER XV

Gated Cardiac Blood Pool Imaging in Acute Myocardial Infarction

Jagmeet S. Soin, M.D.

The technical considerations as well as the clinical applications of multiple gated heart acquisition (MUGA) study of left ventricular function in ambulatory patients have been dealt with in considerable detail in the preceding chapters. Although the assessment of ventricular function with radionuclides is now largely a computer-assisted technique, the earlier dual gated (DUGA) end-diastolic or end-systolic studies were invaluable in the management of patients with acute myocardial infarctions. A great deal of information concerning the cardiac function can be obtained with simple, non-computer based gated cardiac blood pool imaging in a patient who has sustained acute myocardial infarction.

The method used in dual gated imaging to assess left ventricular function has been discussed by Thrall et al. in Chapter 13 of this book. The main advantage of this technique is the simplicity with which the existing nuclear imaging equipment can be adapted to provide cardiac function studies. Generally, the only change required is to interface an electrocardiographic physiological synchronizer to a gamma camera and image recording device. The initial clinical experience with this technique was based on the work performed by Strauss and associates.[1-3] It is now apparent that global and regional ventricular function must be assessed to obtain a comprehensive and objective estimate of the severity of cardiac damage following an acute myocardial infarction. The practical clinical indications for gated cardiac blood pool studies are summarized in Table 15-1.

199

TABLE 15-1
Indications for Gated Cardiac Blood Pool Study in Patients With Acute Myocardial Infarction

1. Detection of acute myocardial infarction.
2. Determination of ejection fraction.
3. Determination of regional ventricular function.
4. Detection of localized abnormalities of ventricular contraction.
5. Separation of pseudoaneurysm from true ventricular aneurysm.
6. Separation of right and left ventricular dysfunction.
7. Detection of pericardial effusion.
8. Evaluation of a new systolic murmur in a patient with acute myocardial infarction.

Clinical Indications

Detection of Acute Myocardial Infarction

Experimental and clinical data have shown that abnormal ventricular contractility promptly ensues following interruption of coronary blood flow.[4] Rigo et al. in a study of 38 patients who had documented acute myocardial infarctions demonstrates that each patient showed abnormal regional ventricular contractility at a site corresponding to the site of infarction. In 36 out of 38 patients definite areas of akinetic tissue were noted. Two patients showed hypokinesis of the affected segment.[5] A representative case is shown in Figure 15-1. This 60-year-old male patient had extensive acute anterior myocardial infarction as shown on a thallium myocardial perfusion study. The corresponding gated blood pool study showed marked akinesis or even dyskinesis of the involved segments. Documentation of regional ventricular contractility has become useful in evaluating patients who have coronary bypass surgery. It is now apparent that at least 4 percent to 10 percent of patients undergoing coronary bypass surgery have acute perioperative myocardial infarctions. The electrocardiogram is frequently nondiagnostic in these patients; however, the combination of serial tests for enzyme changes and ^{99m}Tc (Sn) pyrophosphate scans have a higher sensitivity.[6] The combination of a positive ^{99m}Tc pyrophosphate scan in the same area as the abnormally contracting segment is highly specific for acute myocardial infarction. A scan showing myocardial infarction in a patient who had coronary bypass surgery is shown in Figure 15-2.

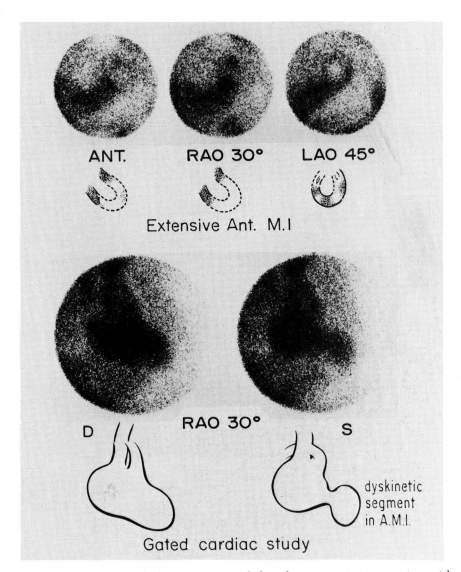

Figure 15-1. Resting thallium-201 myocardial perfusion imaging in a patient with acute myocardial infarction. Note the absence of radioactivity in the anterior apical and inferior walls. The gated blood pool study also identifies the site of myocardial infarction. In addition, it demonstrates dyskinesis associated with acute myocardial infarction and poor ejection fraction.

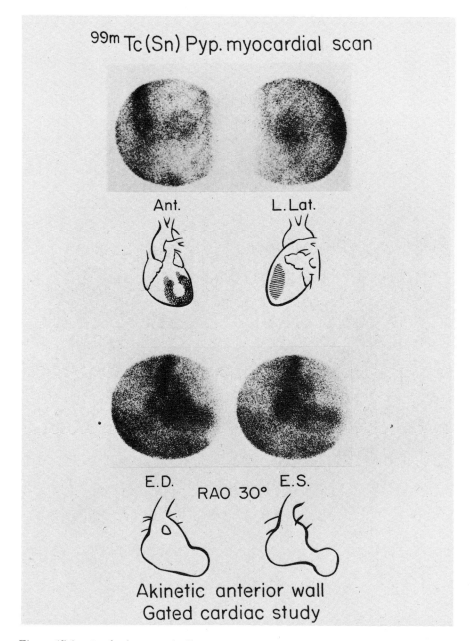

Figure 15-2. Study shows markedly increased uptake in anterior wall of left ventricle in a patient who developed loss of R-wave in precordial leads the fifth day after coronary artery bypass surgery. The gated cardiac blood pool study also demonstrates akinesis of the anterior wall, thus confirming the presence of myocardial infarction.

Determination of Ejection Fraction

The ejection fraction (EF) is the ratio of the left ventricular stroke volume to end-diastolic volume and as a single measurement is considered the best index of total ventricular function.[7] The ejection fraction has been correlated with prognosis in a variety of cardiac disorders.[8,9] Ejection fraction is calculated by measuring the silhouette of the left ventricular cavity as outlined on the end-diastolic and end-systolic images.[2,3] In their early experience, Rigo et al. demonstrated that patients who had acute myocardial infarctions can be divided into three groups on the basis of measured ejection fraction during the early stages of their hospitalization. Group I consisted of patients with slightly reduced ejection fractions, but normal hemodynamic function as indicated by normal systemic blood pressure and cardiac output. Groups II and III consisted of patients with congestive heart failure and cardiogenic shock, respectively. These groups also had progressively compromised ejection fraction values. When the ejection fraction values and extent of regional wall motion abnormalities were correlated, it was noted that the larger the infarction, the lower was the ejection fraction value.[5] It is clear that early mortality during hospitalization is more likely in a patient who shows marked reduction in ejection fraction on admission and no significant improvement after therapy. The extent of myocardial infarction and degree of ejection fraction also affects the prognosis. The incidence of life threatening arrythmias is greater after hospitalization for patients who had poorer ejection fraction values while they were in the hospital.[9]

Detection of Localized Abnormalities in Left Ventricular Contraction

In patients with congestive heart failure following myocardial infarction, the gated blood pool study has been used to differentiate between localized left ventricular aneurysm and diffuse left ventricular hypokinesis. This distinction can be important if any surgical intervention such as coronary revascularization or aneurysectomy is being considered, since patients with diffuse left ventricular hypokinesis have a higher mortality than those with localized aneurysms. In an evaluation of 22 patients who had acute myocardial infarctions followed by congestive heart failure, the gated blood pool scan successfully allowed distinction between those patients with diffuse hypokinesis from those with localized aneurysms. The gated scan was more sensitive an indicator than was abnormal cardiac impulse, S-3 gallop, persistent elevation of ST-T segment on ECG or suspicious plain chest radiograph in the detection of left ventricular aneurysm.[10] Generally, 85 percent of the ventricular aneurysms are associated with anterior myocardial infarctions, and approximately 10 percent of all myocardial infarctions cause aneurysms.[10] Figure 15-3 illustrates a large left ventricular aneurysm which was subsequently resected.

Distinction of Pseudoaneurysm from True Left Ventricular Aneurysm

True aneurysm is a common cause of morbidity in patients who have had acute myocardial infarctions. It is generally formed by the non-contractile myocardial wall in the zone of infarction. The aneurysmal wall is composed of scattered myocardial elements with a matrix of fibrous tissue. It is characteristically a wide-necked, thin wall, poorly contractile pocket that compromises the function of the remaining myocardium. The common complications associated with true aneurysms are left ventricular failure, mural thrombi, or life-threatening arrythmias. Early myocardial rupture is extremely uncommon. A false or pseudoaneurysm is caused by a small contained rupture of the recently infarcted ventricular wall and characteristically it is a large bottle-necked cavity that imparts an hourglass configuration to the venticle. Its wall is composed of an organized hematoma lacking any element of the myocardial wall. Clinically it differs little from true aneurysm except in its tendency to cause late rupture. Previously the only way to make an antemortem diagnosis was by contrast ventriculography. Botvinick, et al. have demonstrated the identifying features of a pseudoaneurysm on the gated cardiac study (Fig. 15-4). It should be emphasized that pseudoaneurysm is a rare complication of acute myocardial infarction, but because of the risk of rupture, early detection and subsequent surgical correction is highly desirable. Its early detection can be aided by employing noninvasive radionuclide studies.[11]

Distinction between Right and Left Ventricular Dysfunction

Heretofore, right ventricular performance could not be evaluated in a patient with coronary artery disease because of the lack of adequate noninvasive techniques. Since its introduction, the gated cardiac blood pool scan in the LAO position has been used to assess the relative size of the right and left ventricles and to determine whether cardiogenic shock is due to right or left ventricular failure. In a study of six patients with cardiogenic shock, three of whom had electrocardiographic evidence of anterior infarction and three had inferior infarctions, the three with anterior myocardial infarctions showed marked left ventricu-

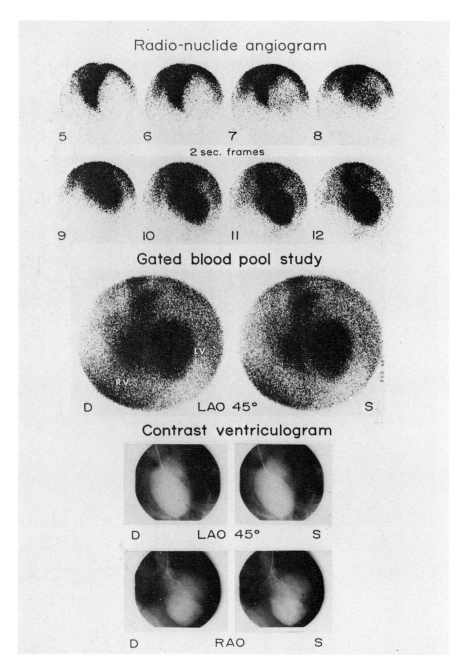

Figure 15-3.   Note how rapid sequence radionuclide angiography can provide information concerning the sizes of right and left ventricle. The gated cardiac images and contrast study demonstrate massive left ventricular aneurysm.

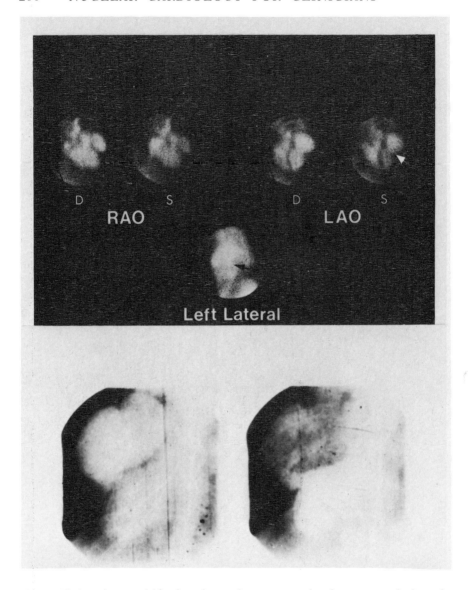

Figure 15-4. This gated blood pool scan demonstrates the characteristic findings for pseudoaneurysm of left ventricle following myocardial infarction (see text). (Courtesy of Dr. E. Botvinick and the American Journal of Cardiology, **37**:1089-1093, 1976).

lar enlargement. In the three with inferior infarctions, the gated cardiac blood pool study revealed right ventricular dilatation and dysfunction. It is now known that therapy for cardiogenic shock due to right ventricular involvement is entirely different from that associated with left ventricular failure. The former responds to volume expansion and has a better prognosis, whereas cardiogenic shock associated with left ventricular dysfunction requires drastic measures such as counterpulsation intra-aortic balloon procedures, pharmaceuticals to maintain systemic blood pressure, or volume restriction.[12] Thus, the gated blood pool study is extremely helpful in making this distinction. Figure 15-5 illustrates this point.

Detection of Pericardial Effusion

Less than 1 percent of patients with acute myocardial infarctions are complicated by cardiac temponade or pericardial effusion. Echocardio-

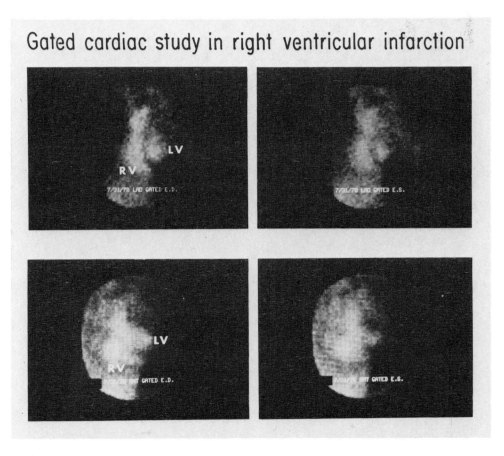

Figure 15-5. Gated cardiac study showing right ventricular enlargement and hypokinesis in a patient with inferior myocardial infarction. Note the normal contractility of the left ventricle. This suggests that inferior myocardial infarction affected the right ventricle only.

graphic techniques remain the first choice for detecting these problems, but on occasion fluid around the heart can be suggested by demonstrating a halo around the cardiac blood pool activity. Care must be exercised to distinguish cases where severe cardiac hypertrophy has caused the same phenomenon.

Evaluation of New Systolic Murmur

A systolic murmur which develops early in the course of acute myocardial infarction should be investigated immediately. The differential diagnosis can be narrowed to the life-threatening rupture of the interventricular septum or of acute mitral regurgitation associated with papillary muscle or rupture of the chordae tendonae. The gated cardiac blood pool studies, especially in conjunction with analysis of the intracardiac transit of a radioactive bolus (radionuclide angiocardiogram), may enable the clinician to exclude the presence of ventricular septal defects. The clinical usefulness of radionuclide studies has not been well documented because of the rarity of these complications, and immediate need for definitive confirmation by cardiac catheterization in order to institute appropriate therapy.

Summary

We have attempted to focus on the role that noninvasive radionuclide techniques can play in the management of patients with cardiac disorders. Needless to say, these techniques are still not fully utilized in the community hospitals. Both computer and non-computer based studies can now be readily available to the clinicians and the cost to benefit ratio can justify the additional expense.[13]

References

1. Strauss, H.W., and Pitt. B.: Evaluation of cardiac function and structure with radioactive tracer techniques. *Circulation* **57**:645-653, 1978.
2. Strauss, H. W., Zaret, B.L., Hurley, P.J., et al.: A scintiphotographic method for measuring left ventricular ejection fraction in man without cardiac catheterization. *Am J Cardiol* **28**:575-580, 1971.
3. Zaret, B.L., Strauss, H. W., Hurley, P.J., et al.: A noninvasive scintiphotographic method for detecting regional ventricular dysfunction in man. *N Engl J Med* **284**:1165-1170,1971.
4. Brooks, H.L., and Gorlin, R.: Pathophysiological basis for abnormal per-

fusion and contraction in coronary artery disease. In Soin, J.S., and Brooks, H.L. (Eds.): *Nuclear Cardiology for Clinicians.* Mt. Kisco, NY, Futura Publishing Co, 1980.

5. Rigo, P., Murray, M., Strauss, H.W., et al.: Left ventricular function in acute myocardial infarction evaluated by gated scintiphotography. *Circulation* **50**:678-684, 1974.

6. Burdine, J. A., Depuey, G.E., Orzan, F., et al.: Scintigraphic, electrocardiographic, and enzymatic diagnosis of perioperative myocardial infarction in patients undergoing coronary artery revascularization. *J Nucl Med* **19**:735, 1978.

7. Cohn, P.F., and Gorlin, R.: Dynamic ventriculography and the role of ejection fraction. *Am J Cardiol* **36**:529-531,1975.

8. Cohn, P.F., Gorlin, R., Cohn, L.H., et al.: Left ventricular ejection fraction as a prognostic guide in surgical treatment of coronary and valvular heart disease. *Am J Cardiol* **34**:136-141, 1974.

9. Schulze, R.A., Rouleau, J., Rigo, P., et al.: Ventricular arrythmias in the late hospital phase of acute myocardial infarction —relation to left ventricular function detected by gated cardiac blood pool scanning. *Circulation* **52**:1006-1011, 1975.

10. Rigo, P., Murray, M., Strauss, H.W., et al.: Scintiphotohraphic evaluation of patients with suspected left ventricular aneurysm. *Circulation* **50**:985-991, 1974.

11. Botvinick, E.H., Shames, D., Hutchinson, J.C., et al.: Noninvasive diagnosis of a false left ventricular aneurysm with radioisotope gated cardiac blood pool imaging—differentiation from true aneurysm. *Am J Cardiol* **37**:1089-1093, 1976.

12. Rigo, P., Murray, M., Taylor, D.R., et al.: Right ventricular dysfunction detected by gated scintiphotography in patients with acute inferior myocardial infarction. *Circulation* **52**:268-273, 1975.

13. Surawicz, B.: How to cope with new technology? The knowledge and the prudence. *Am J Cardiol* **43**:1249-1250, 1979.

CHAPTER XVI

Complementary Role of Echocardiography and Radionuclide Imaging in the Evaluation of Cardiac Anatomy and Function

L. Samuel Wann, M.D., Randolph P. Martin, M.D., Charles M. Gross, M.D., Jagmeet S. Soin, M.D., and Harold L. Brooks, M.D.

During the 1950's and 1960's cardiac catheterization virtually revolutionized the field of cardiac dignosis, particularly following the advent of open heart surgery with its needs for precise preoperative evaluation of cardiac anatomy. Although widely used and generally safe, cardiac catheterization is associated with a small but irreducible risk of significant morbidity and even mortality. For this reason, the decade of the 1970's has been dedicated to the development of noninvasive procedures for the evaluation of cardiac anatomy and function. Two of these newly developed techniques—echocardiography and radionuclide imaging—have met with widespread enthusiasm and are currently available to community hospitals throughout the country.

Principles of Echocardiography

Both M-mode and cross-sectional echocardiography are based on physical principles of pulsed reflected ultrasound. Short bursts or pulses of high frequency sound are produced by an electrically excited crystal applied to the chest wall. These sound waves pass through the chest wall and underlying heart. As the pulses of sound encounter acoustic interfaces, such as the junction between heart muscle and blood, part of the sound passes through the interface, and part is reflected back towards the crystal or transducer, which detects the reflected sound and converts it back into electrical energy for display. This principle is much the same as that of a ray of light striking the surface of a body of water—part of the light is reflected by the surface of the water, creating a mirror-like image, and part of the light passes through the water. As the light passes through the water, it may in turn be reflected by a fish. This second reflection enables us to see the fish within the water. In essence, the use of ultrasound enables us to see through the heart.

M-Mode Echocardiography

M-mode echocardiography uses a single pencil-like beam of ultrasound to examine the heart. This thin beam of sound traverses the intracardiac structures and is reflected by them. When the transducer is not sending out pulses of sound, it detects the reflected beam. The transducer converts these reflected sound waves into electrical energy, and displays them on an oscilloscope. Since the speed of sound transmission through the heart is constant, the distance of a reflecting structure within the heart from the transducer can be calibrated by measuring the time taken for a pulse of sound to travel from the transducer to that structure and return. The distance between two intracardiac structures can thus be appreciated by measuring their relative distances from the ultrasound transducer.

Commonly used ultrasound transducers produce 1000 pulses of sound per second. Each pulse lasts 1/10,000 second, leaving the transducer free to receive reflected sound 99.9 percent of the time. Sound reflected by acoustic interfaces within the heart is displayed on an oscilloscope in the form of small dots. The brightness of each dot represents the strength of the reflection. The distance between the dots is calibrated in centimeters on the vertical axis of the oscilloscope. Since the intracardiac structures represented by this vertical line of dots move with the cardiac cycle, this line of information is swept across the oscilloscope at a constant speed, so that the change in position of an intracardiac structure is represented by the moving line. A strip chart recorder is used to permanently record the oscilloscopic image. Standard records are calibrated in centimeters on the vertical axis and in mm/sec on the horizontal axis. Electrocardiograms and phonocardiograms are commonly recorded simultaneously with the echocardiogram so that cardiac events can be timed throughout the cardiac cycle.

This motion-mode or "M-mode" echocardiogram thus contains information about the vertical position of reflecting interfaces within the thin pencil-like beam of sound, and the movement of these interfaces throughout the cardiac cycle. Intracardiac structures are recognized by their relative positions within this beam, and their characteristic motion patterns during the cardiac cycle. An example of an M-mode echocardiogram of the mitral valve is shown in Figure 16-1. The ultrasound beam first strikes the chest wall, then the right ventricle, the interventricular septum, the left ventricular cavity, the mitral valve leaflets,

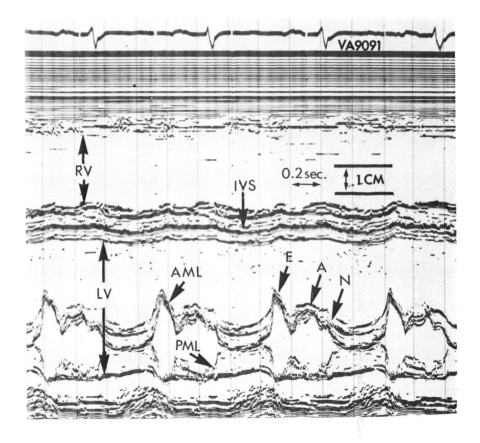

Figure 16-1.   M-mode echocardiogram of the mitral valve. The beam of ultrasound first encounters the chest wall, then the right ventricle (RV), interventricular septum (IVS), left ventricular cavity (LV), anterior mital leaflet (AML) and posterior mitral leaflet (PML). The distance scale in centimeters is indicated on the vertical axis. The interval between two lines represents 0.2 seconds. The mitral leaflets are recognizable by their characteristic M- or W-shaped motion during diastole. The E point or initial opening of the valve is labeled. The A point, which results from atrial systole, can be seen immediately after the P wave on the simultaneous electrocardiogram. In this example the mitral leaflet exhibits a third abnormal movement just prior to closure. This notch (N) results from delayed mitral closure, and is indicative of increased left ventricular end-diastolic pressure.

and the posterior wall of the ventricle. The anterior leaflet of the mitral valve can be recognized by its characteristic M-shaped motion toward the chest wall during diastole. Similarly, the endocardial surfaces of the left ventricle can be recognized by observing motion of these echos toward the center of the left ventricular cavity during systole—the peak of the electrocardiographic R waves. In both these examples it should be emphasized that the motion of a reflecting interface is used to establish its identity. The shape of a structure within the heart is not truly displayed with M-mode echocardiography, since only one dimension is distance. The horizontal axis is time.

Adjacent structures within the heart can be examined by manually angling the thin beam of the ultrasound in different directions (Fig. 16-2). However, distance between laterally placed structures within the heart cannot be measured, and no quantitative spatial orientation is possible. The strength of M-mode echocardiography is its ability to record extremely rapidly occurring events within the heart.

Cross-Sectional Echocardiography

Cross-sectional or two-dimensional echocardiography provides distance information about the location and distance between structures in the lateral as well as vertical dimension. In essence, this is accomplished by rapidly steering the same pencil-like beam of ultrasound used in M-mode echocardiography through an arc. This steering can be accomplished by mechanically moving the transducer, or through an electronic process in which the transducer is not physicaly moved. The transducer again senses sound waves reflected by acoustic interfaces within the heart, and records their distance from the transducer in the axial dimension by measuring the time taken for a pulse of sound to travel to and from a given structure. Distance in the lateral dimension is determined by recording the point within its arc when the beam is encountered by a reflecting interface. Cross-sectional echocardiography images are initially visualized on an oscilloscope. A single frame on the oscilloscope represents one cycle of movement of the ultrasound beam through its arc (Fig. 16-3). The individual precisely spaced vertical lines within this pie-shaped image represent the relative positions of the ultrasound beam as it traverses adjacent areas of the heart. A new frame is created when the beam restarts its cycle through the arc. Sequential frames can be visualized on the oscilloscope in real time or recorded on videotape for later analysis in real time, slow motion or stop-action format. The frame rate or the speed with which new arcs are produced

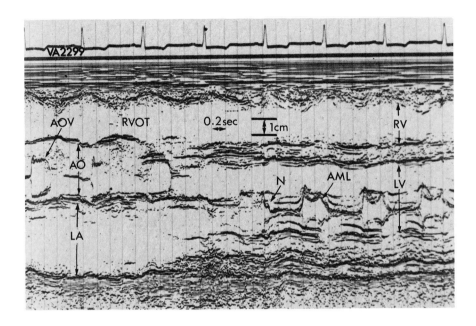

Figure 16-2. M-mode echocardiogram of the aortic and mitral valves. At the left the transducer is directed through the right ventricular outflow tract (RVOT), the aorta (AO) and aortic valve (AVO) and finally the left atrium (LA). A simultaneous electrocardiogram is also recorded. The aortic valve is recognized by its characteristic box-like motion during systole—the valve opens at the peak of the R wave on the electrocardiogram. On the right side of this illustration, the ultrasound transducer has been tilted while continuously recording until it has been directed through the mitral valve. Distance is indicated on the vertical scale, time on the horizontal axis. The aortic and mitral valves are thus viewed sequentially during continous recording to display their relative positions within the heart. However, the lateral (horizontal) distance between these structures cannot be measured. In this example, the aortic valve does not open completely against the walls of the aorta, and the leaflets move toward closure during systole. Both features suggest diminished flow through the valve. A notch (N) similar to that illustrated in Figure 16-1 can be seen on the recording of the mitral valve, and suggests increased left ventricular end-diastolic pressure

determines the ability of cross-sectional echocardiography to resolve motion of intracardiac structures during the cardiac cycle. The frame rate in most systems is 30 per second.

Cross-sectional echocardiography thus produces two-dimensional pie-shaped tomographic images of the heart. Distance between intracardiac structures can be measured in the horizontal as well as vertical axis. Timing of motion is represented as the frame rate. The third dimension

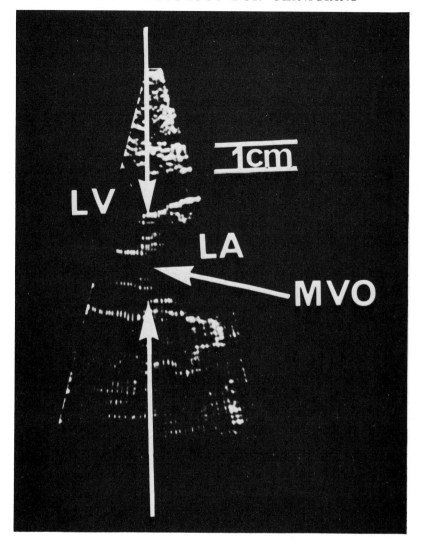

Figure 16-3. Long-axis cross-sectional echocardiogram of a stenotic mitral valve. Images were obtained with a 30-degree mechanical sector scanner. This frame was obtained during early diastole and shows the mitral valve orifice (MVO) as defined by the edges of the anterior and posterior mitral leaflets. Blood flows from the left atrium (LA) through the restricted orifice to the left ventricle (LV) at the left. By twisting the transducer 90 degrees perpendicular to this view, and along the plane defined by the large vertical arrows, a short-axis view of the mitral valve similar to that shown in Figure 16-4 can be obtained. The diameter of the mitral valve orifice can be measured in this long-axis view, while the circumference and area of the orifice can be measured from the short-axis view.

of distance, depth, is not recorded by cross-sectional echocardiography. Each image is in effect a tomographic slice of the heart. In order to examine the entire heart in its three dimensions multiple different slices must be recorded.

Standard Echocardiographic Views

The performance of both M-mode and cross-sectional echocardiograms is limited by the fact that the sound waves do not penetrate bone or air. Thus, the ultrasound transducer must be applied to areas of the body where the ultrasound beam will not strike ribs or lung tissue along its path to the heart. These "acoustic windows" are relatively small and are located in different anatomic sites in different patients, precluding use of pre-set transducer positions to examine individual patients. Standard echocardiographic views are therefore not determined exclusively by external body landmarks, but on the relative positions of the intracardiac structures being visualized.

In Figure 16-1, the standard M-mode echocardiographic view of the mitral valve is defined by the characteristic appearance of the anterior and posterior mitral leaflets opening and closing within the cavity of the left ventricle. This view is usually obtained by placing the ultrasound transducer in the third left intercostal space adjacent to the sternum, but the exact position and angulation of the transducer varies considerably from patient to patient.

Similarly, the "long-axis view of the mitral valve" shown in the cross-sectional echocardiogram in Figure 16-3 is standardized by the characteristic location and appearance of the mitral leaflets and walls of the left ventricle and left atrium. This view is also usually obtained by placing the ultrasound transducer in the third left intercostal space. The transducer is twisted and angled until the arc of ultrasound is aligned parallel with the long-axis of the valve apparatus. This image is a two-dimensional tomogram of the valve—the third dimension, or depth, is absent in this view. In order to examine this third dimension, the operator must twist the transducer 90 degrees until the arc is aligned parallel to the short-axis of the valve. Figure 16-4 is a short-axis, cross-sectional echocardiogram of the mitral valve in a patient with mitral stenosis. This tomographic slice transects the mitral orifice at its narrowest point; the valve area can be measured by planimetering the area of this orifice.

Thus, in order to examine the entire heart with the cross-sectional echocardiographic beam, several transducer positions are used and the transducer is placed in all available acoustical windows. Standard echocardiographic views of the heart are obtained with the transducer on the chest wall transecting various intracardiac structures in both their long- and short-axes. The transducer is also moved to the cardiac apex or subxyphoid area and tilted back in order to transect the heart in its sagittal plane. An "apical four-chamber view" of the heart is shown in

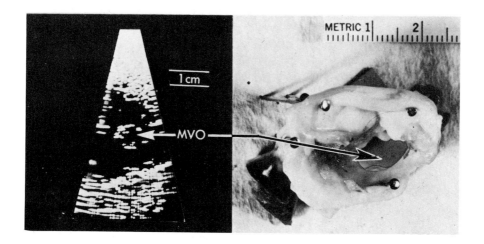

Figure 16-4. (*Left*) Short-axis cross-sectional echocardiogram of a stenotic mitral valve. (*Right*) Surgically excised mitral valve from the same patient shown on the echocardiogram. The mitral orifice appears in the center of the circular left ventricle. Mitral valve area measured both on the echocardiogram and surgical specimen was 1.0 cm².

Figure 16-5. This view is so termed because the transducer is placed at the apex of the heart and positioned such that the arc of sound is directed toward the base of the heart. The cardiac apex, recognized by its characteristic shape and location, is first transected by the beam, followed by the bodies of the left and right ventricles, the mitral and tricuspid valves, and finally the left and right atria. This view is finally standardized by the ultrasound technician who alters the position of the transducer while simultaneously observing the resultant image.

Comparison of Echocardiographic and Nuclear Imaging Techniques

There are several important differences between echocardiography and nuclear imaging:

1. Echocardiography is based on the principle of pulsed, reflected ultrasound. Contrast material need not be injected— the intracardiac structures themselves reflect ultrasound. Nuclear imaging is based on the external detection of ionizing radiation produced by radioactive material injected into the circulation.
2. The quality of echocardiographic examinations are highly dependent on the skill of the operator in properly aligning the ultrasound

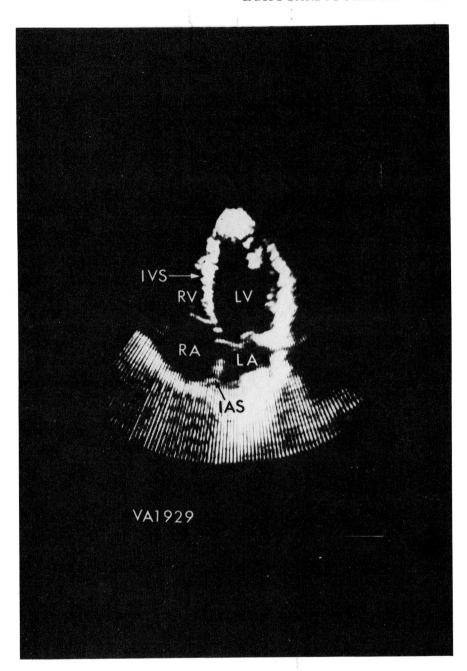

Figure 16-5. Apical four-chamber view of the heart. The transducer is placed directly over the cardiac apex, and tilted so that the arc of ultrasound is directed along a sagittal plane to the base of the heart. All four chambers of the heart can be seen—the right ventricle (RV), left ventricle (LV), right atrium (RA), and left atrium (LA) as well as the interventricular septum (IVS) and interatrial septum (IAS).

transducer. Approximately 10 percent of patients cannot be examined with echocardiography due to the absence of adequate acoustical windows. Nuclear imaging techniques, once operational, are relatively independent of individual operator skill. An adequate examination can be performed in virtually all patients.

3. Echocardiographic views are standardized by the relative positions of intracardiac structures, not necessarily by the location of the transducer on the chest wall. Radionuclide images are standardized by the position of the patient with respect to the camera, such as left anterior oblique or right anterior oblique.

4. Echocardiography does not examine the "whole heart" at one time. M-mode echocardiography detects the motion only with the axial dimension of its slender pencil-like beam. Cross-sectional echocardiography produces real time tomographic images of the heart in two-dimensions. The third dimension is examined sequentially by rotating the transducer, or moving it to another acoustical window. Nuclear imaging techniques detect all radioactivity in a given field. Wall motion is assessed by observing the silhouette of radioactivity within a structure, similar to the cineradiographic detection of injected x-ray contrast material. Global changes in the left ventricle can be assessed by measuring the amount of radioacvitity within the chamber with progression of the cardiac cycle.

5. Echocardiography can detect relatively small intracardiac structures, such as valve leaflets and vegetations. In general, radionuclide techniques do not visualize these small structures.

6. Echocardiography provides excellent resolution of cardiac motion. The pulse repetition rate in M-mode echocardiography is approximately 1000 per second. The frame rate in cross-sectional echocardiography is commonly 30 per second. In general, multiple nuclear images must be gated to the electrocardiogram over several subsequent cardiac cycles in order to resolve cardiac motion with computer reconstruction techniques.

7. Clinical echocardiography is largely limited to the detection and localization of reflecting interfaces within the heart. Characterization of cardiac tissue based on other features of tissue interaction with sound is undergoing investigation. By using such biochemically active radioactive substances as Thallium-201, nuclear imaging can acquire information concerning the cellular function of the heart in a localized area.

Clinical Applications of Echocardiography

M-Mode Echocardiography

Although foreshadowed by the more recently developed technique of cross-sectional echocardiography, M-mode echocardiography continues to be an important means of evaluating cardiac abnormalities. The major strength of M-mode echocardiography is its ability to precisely record the motion of the intracardiac structures transected by its thin beam. The timing and pattern of valve motion is helpful in the diagnosis of such diverse entities as acute aortic regurgitation, mitral stenosis, Ebstein's anomaly, pulmonary hypertension, mitral prolapse, hypertrophic cardiomyopathy and constrictive pericarditis. The relationship of valve motion to pressure and flow continues to be an active area of investigation. Simultaneous recording of valve echograms and phonocardiograms has contributed significantly to our understanding of cardiac physiology.

Chamber dimensions and wall thicknesses are readily measured from M-mode echocardiograms, although in only one dimension. The endocardial surfaces of the normal left ventricle can be seen moving together with systole, and the walls themselves thicken. Areas of ischemia or infarction demonstrate abnormal motion, and the walls may fail to thicken normally or even become thinner with systole. Even small changes in wall motion caused by conduction disturbances such as Wolf-Parkinson-White syndrome and bundle branch blocks can be detected.

A qualitative appreciation of the overall internal anatomy of the heart can be gained by scanning the ultrasound transducer sequentially through adjacent intracardiac structures. Many of the anatomic deformities of congenital heart disease can be recognized with M-mode echocardiography, and areas of segmental wall motion abnormalities can be appreciated in patients with ischemic heart disease. However, M-mode echocardiography is limited because it does not offer true spatial orientation of cardiac structures.

Cross-Sectional Echocardiography

Although sacrificing some of the time resolution afforded by M-mode echocardiography, cross-sectional echocardiography offers the advantage of two-dimensional imaging. A series of tomographic images in mutually orthagonal planes can delineate the size and shape of the heart and intracardiac structures. By recording short-axis views of the mitral valve, the actual area of the mitral orifice can be measured in patients with mitral stenosis. Similarly, the diameter of aortic valve opening can be measured in patients with aortic stenosis, helping to quantitate the severity of obstruction. The size, shape, location and mobility of cardiac masses, including tumors, thrombi and vegetations can be readily appreciated with cross-sectional echocardiography.

Evaluation of wall motion abnormalities in patients with ischemic heart disease is an especially important application of cross-sectional echocardiography. The spatially oriented real time images greatly facilitate observation of ventricular aneurysms and segmental dysynergy. Cross-sectional echocardiography and left ventricular cineangiography usually correlate well, although disagreements do exist because of the fundamental differences in imaging techniques and errors among observers. The two-dimensional images produced by cross-sectional echocardiography also facilitate the recognition of structural abnormalities encountered in congenital heart disease.

In general, the improved spatial orientation of cross-sectional echocardiography allows recognition of cardiac anatomy based on the size, shape, location and movement of sound reflecting interfaces within the heart. Cross-sectional echocardiography does not, however, allow simultaneous visualization of the entire heart. Numerous tomographic slices must be integrated in order to appreciate the global structure and function of the heart.

Comparison of the Clinical Applications of Echocardiography and Nuclear Imaging

Table 16-1 lists a number of potential applications of echocardiography, nuclear imaging and cardiac catheterization together with an arbitrary estimation of the clinical usefullness of each procedure. These designations are based on our experience, and may be subject to debate. In general, echocardiography is superior to nuclear imaging in the evaluation of valvular heart disease because of its ability to directly visualize the valves. In addition, echocardiography is probably the procedure of choice for the evaluation of IHSS, left atrail myxoma, valvular vegetations and pericardial effusions.

Radionuclide imaging of the left ventricle is superior to echocardiography because images can be made of virtually all patients, even during exercise, and the resultant images are readily quantitated. The measurement of radionuclide ejection fraction is particularly attractive

TABLE 16-1

Comparative Usefulness of Cardiac Catheterization, Nuclear Imaging and Echocardiography

	Cardiac Catheterization	Nuclear Imaging	M-Mode Echocardiography	Cross-Sectional Echocardiography
Mitral stenosis	++	−	+	++
Mitral regurgitation	+	(+)°	±	(+)°
Mitral prolapse	+	−	+	(++)°
Aortic stenosis	++	(+)°	±	+
Aortic regurgitation	+	(++)°	+	(+)°
IHSS	++	++	++	++
Tricuspid stenosis	+	−	±	(+)°
Tricuspid regurgitation	±	−	−	(+)°
Pulmonary stenosis	++	−	+	(++)°
Left atrial myxoma	+	(+)°	++	++
Valvular vegetations	−	−	+	++
Intracardiac shunts	++	+	+	(++)°
Pericardial effusion	±	+/−	++	++
Pulmonary hypertension	++	−	(+)°	−
Intracardiac thrombi	+	−	−	(++)°
Direct visualization of LV walls	−	−	+	++
Detection of segmental LV dysfunction	++	++	++	++
LV ejection fraction	+	++	±	±
LV aneurysm	++	++	±	++
Coronary artery anatomy	++	−	−	(+)°
Coronary flow	(+)°	(+)°	−	−
Myocardial perfusion	−	++	−	−
LV dysfunction with exercise	+	++	−	(+)°
Cardiac output	++	(+)°	(+)°	(+)°

++ Excellent, + Good, − Poor or no application, ° Investigational because of its independence of left ventricular geometery. Radioactivity within the left ventricular cavity can be measured throughout the cardiac cycle. The ejection fraction can be calculated without tracing the limits of the left ventricular walls, and without measuring absolute volume. Echocardiography provides better resolution of rapidly occurring events than does nuclear imaging, but requires multiple views to examine the entire ventricle, and calculation of such global indices as ejection fraction are dependent on the complex internal geometry of the left ventricle. Nuclear imaging alo has the advantage of using metabolically active tracer agents to assess myocardial perfusion.

Conclusions

Echocardiography and nuclear imaging are both new techniques which have significantly improved our ability to noninvasively assess the functional anatomy of the heart. These procedures are still evolving rapidly, and their final applications in most areas of clinical heart disease have not been established. Few studies have been performed comparing the relative sensitivity, specificity and overall effectiveness of each technique for a given clinical entity.

Echocardiography and nuclear imaging are technically dissimilar, and the images of the heart are fundamentally different and not directly comparable. Echocardiography is unique in its direct visualization of the interior structures of the heart, but is hampered by the fact that adequate studies cannot be done in approximately 10 percent of patients. The major advantage of nuclear imaging is it applicability to virtually all patients, even during exercise, and the ability to employ biologically active radiopharmaceuticals for cardiac imaging.

Table 16-2 lists several features of an ideal cardiac diagnostic procedure, together with an estimation of how closely cardiac catheterization, nuclear imaging and echocardiography meet these objectives. Clearly, none of these techniques is "ideal." One procedure complements the other. The choice of an individual diagnostic procedure will depend largely on the pathologic entity suspected, and the vigor with which the clinician wishes to pursue an evaluation. It seems reasonable to state that echocardiography is the preferred technique for noninvasive evaluation of valvular and congenital heart disease, while nuclear imaging is superior in the assessment of global left ventricular function and for the detection of regional ischemia. The relative roles of echocardiography and nuclear imaging in the assessment of segmental wall motion have not been established.

TABLE 16-2
Comparison of Cardiac Catheterization, Nuclear Imaging and Echocardiography

Features of an Ideal Diagnostic Procedure	Cardiac Catheterization	Nuclear Imaging	Echocardiography
Low risk	—	++	++
Painless	—	++	++
Noninvasive	—	++	++
No patient cooperation (including respiration and rhythm)	—	±	—
Little operator skill	—	+	—
Easily repeatable	—	++	++
Portable	—	+	++
Available in emergencies	—	—	++
No interference with cardiac physiology	—	++	++
High time resolution	+	+	++
Data output readily quantitated	+	++	±
Technically adequate study possible in all patients	+	++	—

— Poor
+ Good
++ Excellent

Echocardiography and nuclear imaging should be viewed as complementary rather than competitive procedures. Each technique has its strengths and weaknesses. Employed together, these procedures greatly improve the clinician's ability to evaluate patients with heart disease.

References

1. Well, P.N.T.: *Physical Principles of Ultrasonic Diagnosis.* Academic Press, New York, 1969.
2. Feigenbaum, H.: *Echocardiography.* Lea and Febiger, Philadelphia, 1976.
3. Nanda, N.C., and Gramiak, R.: *Clinical Echocardiography.* C.V. Mosby, St. Louis, 1978.
4. Popp, R.L.: Echocardiographic evaluation of left ventricular function. *N Engl J Med* **296**:856-858, 1977.
5. Weyman, A.E., and Feigenbaum, H.: Symposium on echocardiography. *Am J Med* **62**:799-804, 1977.

CHAPTER XVII

Nuclear Cardiology in Congenital Heart Disease

Philip O. Alderson, M.D.

Congenital heart disease is present in less than 1 percent of babies surviving at birth,[1] but these children often have long and complicated courses of medical and surgical therapy. For this reason noninvasive radionuclide techniques, with a low radiation dose, can provide a valuable means for diagnosing and monitoring their cardiac condition. This chapter will emphasize the utility of these techniques in diagnosing cardiac shunts and evaluating left ventricular function.

Left-To-Right Cardiac Shunts

The most common congenital heart abnormalities are ventricular septal defect (VSD), atrial septal defect (secundum type) (ASD), and patent ductus arteriosus (PDA).[1] When these defects are present, blood in the right and left sides of the heart will be mixed. The pattern of flow across the defect is determined by the relation of right- and left-sided pressures during the cardiac cycle. Many defects are associated with both left-to-right (L-R) flow and right-to-left (R-L) shunt flow during different phases of the cardiac cycle.[2] Usually the net effect of the shunt is unidirectional, and the defects are labelled either L-R or R-L shunts.

Technique

Radionuclide angiocardiography begins with the child lying supine beneath a gamma camera equipped with a high sensitivity collimator. The patient is given a bolus injection of radionuclide, usually ^{99m}Tc-pertechnetate or ^{99m}Tc-DTPA chelate. The tracer must arrive in the lungs as a discrete, short bolus (2.5 sec.) if the amount of shunting is to be assessed accurately. In our experience a good bolus may be injected most successfuly with a saline flush to propel a small volume (0.5 cc) of radiotracer. In infants the best vein to inject is the external jugular vein. Veins in the antecubital fossa may also be suitable. The basilic vein, which is located in the medial portion of the antecubital fossa, usually provides the most direct route to the heart. The arm should be extended during injection to minimize venous tortuosity in the axillary region. Before the injection patency of the vein should be checked by injecting a 1 to 2 cc test dose of saline. Just before injection, the position of the patient under the camera should be rechecked using a radioactive source marker. It is especially important to re-evaluate patient position when children are studied, as they frequently move partially out of the field of view, during the final preparation for injection. If the patient is so large that the whole thorax cannot be viewed at once, the patient should be positioned so the right lung is fully visualized. In most patients the heart and great vessels obscure a large portion of the left lung, and the right lung is the most useful region of interest.

Left-to-right shunts can often be detected on serial images taken during the initial cardiopulmonary transit of the tracer.[3,4] A series of images are taken at 0.5 to 1-second intervals while the patient lies supine beneath the gamma camera. Normally the radionuclide activity appears first in the superior vena cava, then in the right side of the heart, next in the lungs, then in the left ventricle, and finally in the aorta. Shortly after the appearance of activity in the aorta, activity in the lung ceases. In a patient with left-to-right shunt (L-R), the sequence appears normal until the aortic phase. Activity persists in the lungs after the tracer reaches the aorta because part of the tracer in the left ventricle is pumped back into the lungs via the L-R shunt. Careful inspection of the images may help differentiate an intracardiac L-R shunt like an ASD or VSD from an extracardiac PDA. In patients with intracardiac shunts the circulation is abnormal in the early phases of the cardiac cycle, thus the right side of the heart shows activity. Since a PDA returns activity directly to a pulmonary artery from the aorta, this "smudging" of intracardiac activity is absent, and the right heart is void of activity during shunt re-circulation.

Although imaging is useful in evaluating L-R shunts, advances have been made because radionuclide methods can quantitate R-L shunts accurately and reproducibly. Folse and Braunwald[5] demonstrated in 1962 that radioactive tracers could be used to evaluate the cause of a heart murmur and to diagnose a L-R shunt. Their technique was based on monitoring the pulmonary time-activity curve after the intravenous injection of radioactive tracer. They used a simple count ratio

(C2/C1 ratio) to indicate the presence of a L-R shunt; C1 is the count rate at the point on the descending limb which occurs at the time T2=2×T1. The count ratio (C2/C1) method has been used widely [6-9] and can discriminate normal patients from those with shunts or other types of heart disease. The method has not been as reliable for distinguishing between patients with shunts and those with other abnormalities such as valvular heart disease.

Recently improved technology has allowed the size of shunts to be determined on the basis of changes in the area under the pulmonary time-activity curve (rather than the value of two points of the curve). Two methods have been used, and both require mathematical curve fitting to the data in the pulmonary time-activity curve. Anderson et al.[10] suggested dividing the outflow portion of the pulmonary time-activity curve into two sections by extending an exponential function from its peak. The area under the time-activity curve is divided into two regions, one above the extrapolated line (area "X") and one below it (area "Y") (Fig. 17-1A). The ratio of these areas (X/Y area ratio) is used to determine the presence and size of a shunt. The gamma function method of Maltz and Treves[11] uses a computer to help fit the gamma variate function to the initial pulmonary transit. This function is then extrapolated to the baseline. The difference between the area under this curve (A_1) and the real data curve is small in patients without shunts. When a difference does exist, a second gamma function is fitted to the difference (Fig. 17-1B), and the ratio of this area (A_2) and the initial area (A_1) is used to quantitate the shunt as:

$$QP/QS = \frac{A}{A_1 - A_2}$$

The accuracy of the C2/C1 ratio method and of these area ratio techniques has been systematically compared in the population of 50 children suspected of having cardiac shunts.[12] Shunts with an oximetry ratio of greater than 1.2:1 were detected by both area ratio methods and the C2/C1 method. Some shunts of less than 1.2:1 were detected, but results were inconsistent at this level for all methods. When the C2/C1 ratio was used, half the patients who had heart disease but no shunt were either falsely classified or classified as borderline abnormal (Fig. 17-2). In addition, one normal child had a C2/C1 ratio that was borderline abnormal. This lack of specificity is a major disadvantage of the C2/C1 approach. Both area ratio techniques showed greater specificity in this same patient population. The gamma function technique provided the best discrimination and had the best correlation and lowest standard error when compared with the results of shunt size determination by oximetry (Table 17-1).

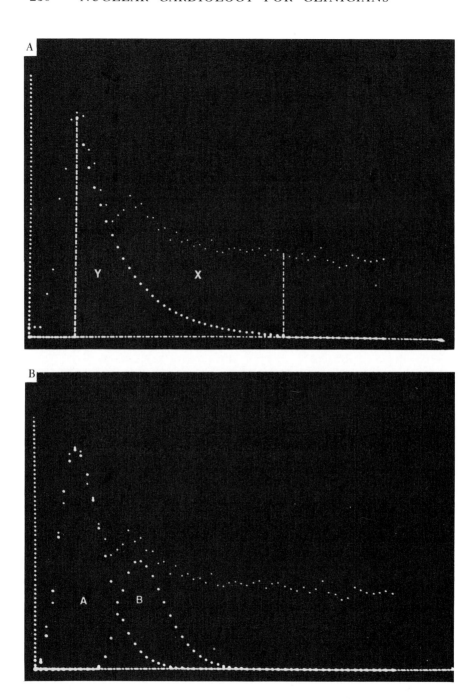

Figure 17-1.   The pulmonary time-activity curve of a child with a 2:1 L-R cardiac shunt is shown. In *A* the curve has been fitted by the exponential method. In *B* the same curve has been fitted by the gamma function method. (See text for discussion.)

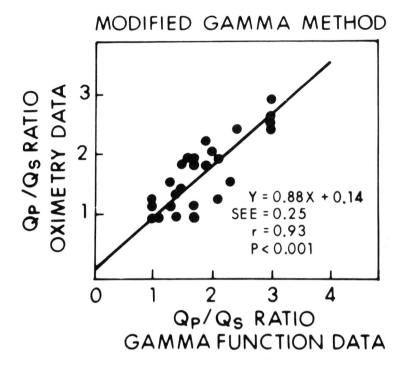

Figure 17-2. The relationship between QP/QS calculated by oximetry and the gamma function method is shown. These results were obtained in studies of 50 children with suspected L-R shunts. There are less than 50 dots in the graph because some patients had the same QP/QS.

Gamma Function Validation

The accuracy and reproducibility of the gamma function method for quantitating L-R cardiac shunts has been investigated in dogs with surgically created chronic, stable ASDs.[13] Each of the eleven such dogs with a surgically created ASD had one radionuclide angiocardiogram. The examinations were performed on ten different days, evenly spaced

TABLE 17-1
Comparison of Radionuclide and Oximetry Determination of Shunt Size°

Method	Shunts only (n = 30)	All Patients (n = 50)
C_2/C_1 Ratio	0.76 (± 0.40)	0.84 (± 0.34)
Exponential fit	0.84 (± 0.33)	0.86 (± 0.33)
Gamma function	0.86 (± 0.29)	0.93 (± 0.25)

°Values given are correlation coefficient ± standard error of estimate.

over a three-week period (Table 17-2). The coefficient of variation for 110 measurements in the 11 dogs was 11.2 percent. The reproducibility of several shunt size measurements performed on the same day was even better than those obtained in the day-to-day studies. A total of 20 measurements were made in five dogs, using computer subtraction between trials to remove interference caused by background counts remaining from previous injections. In these studies the standard deviation ranged between 5.6 and 7.4 percent of the shunt size measured, and the coefficient of variation of the 20 measurements was 7.0 percent. These results show that quantitative radionuclide angiocardiography using the gamma function method is reproducible, and thus is a suitable technique for serial measurements of shunt size.

TABLE 17-2

Reproducibility of Radioangiocardiographic Shunt Determinations in Experimental ASD

Dog No.	QP/QS Ratio ($\pm$ SD)	Percent SD
1	1.56 $\pm$ 0.14	9.0
2	1.70 $\pm$ 0.18	10.6
3	1.69 $\pm$ 0.24	14.2
4	1.86 $\pm$ 0.18	9.7
5	1.72 $\pm$ 0.17	9.9
6	1.56 $\pm$ 0.19	12.2
7	1.76 $\pm$ 0.22	12.5
8	1.68 $\pm$ 0.23	13.7
9	1.45 $\pm$ 0.13	9.0
10	1.71 $\pm$ 0.23	13.4
11	1.69 $\pm$ 0.20	11.8

This animal model also allowed testing of the gamma function method against direct measurements of aortic and pulmonary flow made by electromagnetic flow probes. Three to nine months after the atrial septal defect had been created surgically, seven animals underwent successful banding of the pulmonary outflow tract. In one animal a snare was placed on the ascending aorta to create a supravalvular aortic obstruction. These maneuvers provided shunt sizes which spanned the clinical useful range from 1:1 to 3:1. There was close agreement between the shunt size determinations made by the flow probes and the gamma function technique (Fig. 17-3).

These experiments emphasize the functional nature of shunt meas-

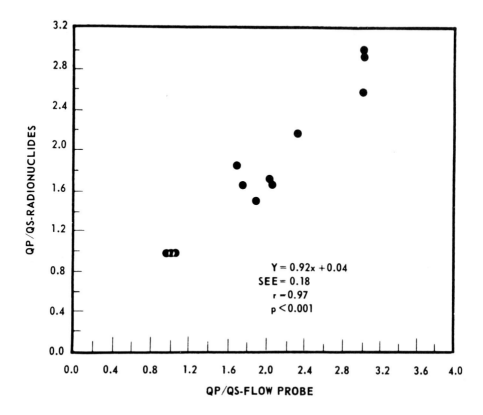

Figure 17-3. The relationship between QP/QS calculated by the gamma function method and electromagnetic flow probes in dogs with atrial septal defects is shown.

urements derived from pulmonary time-activity curves. After the pulmonary outflow tracts were banded, right heart pressures were elevated and the left-to-right shunt actually disappeared, and QP/QS was 1.0 as determined by both flow probes and the gamma function techniques. In one animal with the partial aortic obstruction, the opposite effect was seen. Aortic obstruction raised left heart pressures and augmented the left-to-right component of the ASD shunt. Flow probes and the gamma function showed a large L-R shunt during this phase of the experiment. Thus, the pulmonary time-activity curve reflected the hemodynamic significance of the shunt, which could be changed physiologically with altering the size of the ASD. This means that a QP/QS of 1.0 by radionuclide angiocardiography can not exclude an anatomic septal defect in the presence of pulmonary stenosis. However, a QP/QS of 1.0 does effectively exclude a L-R shunt of hemodynamic significance.

Clinical Utility

Results of the gamma function method have been reported for over 150 patients [12,14] and the correlation with oximetry determinations of shunt size has been excellent (r=0.93) (Fig. 17-2). The useful range for shunt size quantitation is Qp/QS = 1.2 to 3.0. The technique has been useful for quantitating L-R shunt size in patients with atrial or ventricular septal defects, a patent ductus arteriosus, or combinations of these lesions. Patent ductus arteriosus (PDA) often has a characteristic appearance. Since PDA is an extracardiac shunt, there is no abnormal flow within the heart; and the right side of the heart is devoid of radionuclide activity during the early phase of the shunt recirculation. In addition, pulmonary shunt flow is often asymmetric, with the larger QP/QS ratio usually in the left lung. Thus, the combination of a normal recirculation in the right side of the heart and asymmetric shunting to the pulmonary artery, strongly suggests a PDA. When an asymmetric shunt is present, the average QP/QS is usually reported. Askenazi et al.[14] studied 16 patients with L-R shunts that had either pulmonic stenosis or had undergone pulmonary banding. There was excellent agreement between shunt size measured by the gamma function algorithm and oximetry. These results confirm the experimental evidence that the QP/QS gamma function ratio is a good monitor of the hemodynamic significance of a L-R shunt.

The test may be used in numerous clinical situations: (1) to investigate children with a heart murmur of uncertain origin; (2) to follow children with small L-R shunts that may close without surgery; (3) to separate cardiac from pulmonary disease in infants; and (4) to follow children after surgical repair or palliation of congenital heart disease (e.g., to determine the functional status of Glenn Shunt or Mustard operation). The radiation dose delivered to a child during the procedure is in order of magnitude less than that received during cardiac angiography, and the radionuclide study hardly ever requires sedation. Judicious use of the technique can thus help avoid cardiac catheterization and angiography in some children.

Right-To-Left Cardiac Shunts

The cyanotic child with congenital heart disease usually has a right-to-left (R-L) cardiac shunt. Surgery is often required to correct or palliate tetralogy of Fallot or similar abnormalities. Preoperative cardiac catheterization is the most common diagnostic procedure and oxygen saturation measurements are used to quantitate the magnitude of shunting.

Radionuclide studies can be used to screen patients for catheterization and to monitor their clinical course, especially after palliative surgery. Radionuclide angiocardiography with ^{99m}Tc-pertechnetate can be used to detect R-L shunts by the altered flow patterns.[3,4] The left ventricle and/or aorta appear too early during the flow sequence, and are visualized as, or even before, the radiotracer arrives in the lungs. R-L shunts can be quantified using ^{99m}Tc-pertechnetate,[15] but the most widely used radionuclide method for quantifying the size of a R-L shunt uses ^{99m}Tc-labeled lung scanning particles.[16] After these particles are injected intravenously, the partition of activity between the systemic circulation and the lungs is determined. If no R-L shunt is present, some of the radiolabeled particles will pass through the shunt to be distributed throughout the systemic circulation, including the kidneys, brain, and other organs. If activity is seen in the kidneys, the shunt is usually greater than 15 percent.

The exact magnitude of the R-L shunt can be determined by quantifying the whole-body distribution of activity together with the pulmonary net counts:

$$\% \text{ R-L Shunt} = \frac{\text{Total Body Count - Total Lung Count}}{\text{Total Body Count}}$$

Gates et al.[16] studied 24 children with R-L shunts using this method. Six studies were unsatisfactory because of poor cooperation by the children (crying may alter the shunt size) or poor particle preparations. The correlation between the size of the R-L shunt as determined by the tracer method and standard Fick calculations was good (r=0.79) in the remaining 18 patients. Early measurement of the particle distribution is important. If fragmentation of the tracer particles occurs or the radiopharmaceutical is metabolized, systemic activity may be spuriously elevated. Although these studies have been performed without complications in many children, caution is advised because the technique results in embolization of systemic and end-arteries. We recommend that the total number of injected particles be restricted to a 70,000-100,000 maximum.

Ventricular Dysfunction

Left Ventricle

Children with many types of congenital heart disease are now surviving into adolescence and adulthood. This improved life expectancy can be traced largely to the introduction, roughly twenty years ago, of open heart surgery for palliation or correction of these diseases. Since many of these children continue to have signs or symptoms of cardiac dysfunction, a reliable, noninvasive, and safe technique like radionuclide imaging should be useful for evaluating and quantifying left ventricular performance. The only risk associated with these radionuclide studies is the minimal radiation exposure. The whole-body exposure from a dose of ^{99m}Tc-pertechnetate is 0.01 to 0.02 rad/mCi. Technetium-99m labeled human serum albumin (Tc-HSA) also gives a whole-body dose of 0.01 to 0.02 rad/mCi and a blood dose of 0.05 rad/mCi. The radiation doses received in these studies are all below those specified as safe by the FDA (i.e., 10 percent of the specified adult dose).

Gated blood pool imaging and ventricular function studies have been used more widely in adults than in children, and these techniques are described in detail elsewhere in this text. These studies have been used to determine ejection fraction and regional wall motion in children,[18] and they will almost certainly be more widely used in the future. The studies are performed after equilibration of ^{99m}Tc-HSA or red blood cells (215 μCi/Kg) in the vascular compartment. Patients lie supine beneath a gamma camera fitted with a low energy, "all purpose" parallel hole collimator placed in the 40° left anterior oblique (LAO) projection. When infants are studied, a converging collimator should be used. Electrocardiographic leads are attached to the child in standard fashion, and data are acquired continuously in synchrony with the electrocardiogram. Acquisition time is approximately 15 minutes. For image display, data from several hundred cardiac cycles, partitioned into 14 to 16 frames per cycle, are added to give images of good statistical quality. These images are then displayed as a continuous movie to allow evaluation of regional wall motion. These cinematic studies show close agreement with angiographic measurements of ejection fraction and wall motion.[19]

We have found these studies useful in evaluating response of the left ventricle to exercise. Exercise studies in children present several unique problems. First, young children are usually unwilling subjects and will not perform sustained supine bicycle exercise. In addition, many current model supine bicycles must be attached near the end of the scanning table. Modifications are necessary so children with short legs can reach the pedals. We have performed exercise ventricular function studies in children receiving the cardiotoxic chemotherapeutic agent adriamycin. Our patients receiving low doses of adriamycin have not suffered adverse cardiac responses. Children have had as many as five serial ventricular function studies over a two-year period, and the ejection fraction values have varied less than 5 percent. We have also performed paried rest-exercise studies in children with cystic fibrosis (unpublished data). Only three of twenty children had abnormal LV functions at rest. Each of these children had severe pulmonary disease. Two of eight children with normal LV function at rest showed a decreased ejection fraction with exercise. These children had moderately severe lung disease. The findings demonstrate that some children with cystic fibrosis have LV dysfunction, and that for a few of these children the condition will be correctly diagnosed only during exercise studies. Neither cystic fibrosis or adriamycin toxicity are usually described as types of congenital heart disease, but experiences with these children indicate the feasibility of paired rest-exercise studies in children. These methods will almost certainly be applied in the long-term evaluation of children with congenital cardiac anomalies.

Right Ventricle

Some types of congenital heart disease affect primarily the right ventricle (RV). This may occur with any type of pulmonic stenosis, or secondary to chronic RV overload from a large L-R shunt. A large L-R shunt can also lead to pulmonary hypertension and secondary RV strain with reversal of the shunt to a R-L direction (Eisenmenger complex). In the Ebstein anomaly a prolapsed tricuspid valve causes "atrialization" of a portion of the RV and several diseases affecting the right side of the heart usually result. Congenital heart diseases of the lung such as cystic fibrosis can also cause right heart strain. In any of these situations a noninvasive technique for quantifying RV function would be useful. Because of problems with RV geometry and difficulties in background selection, standard blood pool techniques cannot be applied to the RV. Currently the RV is best approached by obtaining a beat-to-beat ejection fraction during the first transit of a bolus of tracer through the RV. An instrument that is particularly well-suited to these studies is the multicrystal gamma camera (Baird-Atomic).[20] This machine can acquire high count data rapidly during the first transit because its multicrystal array minimizes dead-time count loss (see Chapter 4). The study of Steele et al.[21] compared RV beat to beat determinations of ejection fraction with biplane contrast angiography, and found a significant correlation (r=0.85, p .01). These techniques have not yet been widely applied to congenital heart disease, but several groups are evaluating RV function in children with cystic fibrosis (CF). In our CF population of 20 children, nine had a right ventricle ejection fraction (RVEF) which was more than two standard deviations below normal. The eventual impact of the multicrystal camera on studies of RV function depends, to a large extent, on whether first-pass techniques with the Anger camera[22,23] become widely used for quantifying RV function.

Valvular Heart Disease

Congenital valvular heart disease usually occurs in association with other cardiac anomalies, but may occur as an isolated abnormality.[1] Aortic stenosis is more common than aortic insufficiency, but mitral insufficiency is more common than mitral stenosis. Mitral insufficiency is commonly associated with corrected transposition of the great vessels, endocardial fibroelastosis, aberrant left coronary artery, or the Marfan syndrome. Any of these valvular abnormalities can also occur secondary to acquired rheumatic heart disease.

Evaluation of the severity of aortic and mitral regurgitation has proven difficult.[24] We developed a simple technique for measuring valvular regurgitation based on gated cardiac blood pool scans.[25] The images are performed in the left anterior oblique 45° projection and provide simultaneous visualization of the left and right ventricles. Measurement of the change in counts over the right and left ventricles reflects their respective total stroke volume variations, and a ratio of these counts changes (stroke indices) can be calculated. In normal individuals the right ventricular stroke volume is equal to the left ventricular stroke volume, and the left-to-right stroke index ratio is near unity. Regions of interest are drawn over the left and right ventricles, and the change in counts in each ventricular area between systole and diastole is determined. The results are expressed as a ratio of the change in counts in the left ventricular area over the change in counts in the right ventricular area (LV/RV stoke index ratio). This ratio ($\frac{X}{1}$) can be transformed to express the regurgitant fraction ($\frac{X-1}{X}$) as a frequent mode of quantification of valvular regurgitation. In 26 patients with valvular regurgitation, the mean ratio was 2.44 (range 1.36 to 5.30). Among the 30 patients studied by cardiac catheterization, the largest ratios were observed in three of the 12 patients with isolated mitral regurgitation (4.61, 5.20, 5.30). Four patients had isolated aortic regurgitations; the largest LV/RV stroke ratio in this group was 2.86. The good agreement between angiographic grading and the LV/RV stroke ratio is shown in Figure 17-4.

While our study limited use of the stroke index to valvular insufficiency, the concept may have wider applicability. Comparison of the right and left ventricular stroke index could be applied to other lesions

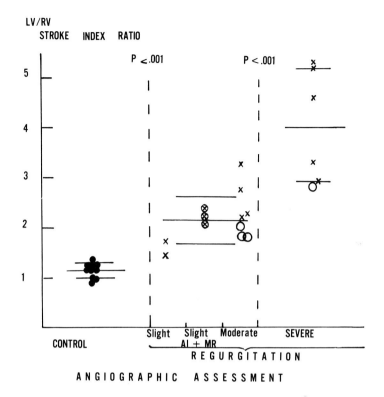

Figure 17-4. The relationship between LV/RV stroke ratio and an independent angiographic grading of valvular insufficiency is shown. The differences between controls, patients with mild-to-moderate insufficiency and those with severe insufficiency are highly significant (p. < .001).

that overload only one ventricle, whether right or left. Measurement of the stroke index ratio might thus be used to estimate right-sided valvular regurgitation, unidirectional shunts and the relative output of each circuit in complete transposition of the great vessels. The greatest advantage of the technique is it simplicity. Virtually any nuclear medicine facility that can acquire gated cardiac studies can apply the technique. It does not require complex data processing. Although further validation of the technique is needed, the initial clinical results with mitral and aortic regurgitation suggest that the technique can detect and estimate regurgitant flow.

Myocardial Abnormalities

Congenital myocardial abnormalities can be evaluated with thallium-201, a tracer which enters viable, perfused myocardial cells as a potassium analog. Congenital myocardial anomalies are rare. One such abnormality which has been investigated by ^{201}Tl imaging is the single ventricle. In this condition, which accounts for 2 to 3 percent of all congenital heart disease,[1] the interventricular septum fails to develop. This condition is often difficult to differentiate from severe tetralogy of Fallot, since both are characterized by cyanosis and cardiomegaly. Strauss et al.[26] have demonstrated that ^{201}Tl imaging will clearly delineate the ventricular septum even if it contains a large septal defect. Patients with a single ventricle will show just one large ventricular cavity. Thus, contrast angiography is not required to make this diagnosis in some children.

Thallium-201 imaging has also been used in children suspected of having anomalous left coronary artery arising from the left pulmonary artery (D. Gilday, personal communication). These children usually present in infancy with cardiomegaly, tachycardia, and episodes of diaphoresis, and may have an electrocardiogram suggesting myocardial infarction. This is a potentially lethal abnormality. Most of these children die unless they have excellent coronary collaterals. Fortunately, these patients respond well to coronary artery surgery,[1] so it is important to diagnose this problem before irreparable damage occurs. Thallium-201 imaging demonstrates perfusion defects in these patients. An abnormal ^{201}Tl study in a child suspected of having this problem is a clear indication for coronary angiography.

Summary

Nuclear cardiology provides a convenient, safe, low-risk means of evaluating a variety of congenital heart abnormalities. Cardiac shunts can be detected and measured, and serial follow-up examinations can be done with good reproducibility. Left and right ventricular function can be analyzed on a global and regional basis, and ventricular performance at rest and during exercise can be evaluated. In addition, the severity of valvular regurgitation can be measured, and myocardial anomalies can be imaged with [201]Tl. The radiation exposure from these procedures is low, especially when compared to doses received during cardiac catheterization and angiography. Thus, for the child with congenital heart disease, nuclear cardiology represents an excellent means of screening and follow-up evaluation after therapy.

References

1. Friedberg, C.K.: Congenital heart disease. In *Diseases of the Heart*, 3rd Ed. W.B. Saunders, Philadelphia, 1966, pp. 1187-1311.

2. Alexander, J.A., Rembert, J.C., Sealy, W.C., et al.: Shunt dynamics in experimental atrial septal defects. *J Appl Physiol* 39:281-286, 1975.

3. Stocker, F.P., Kinser, J., Weber, J.W., et al.: Pediatric radioangiocardiography: Shunt diagnosis. *Circulation* 47:819-826, 1973.

4. Kriss, J.P., Enright, L.P., Hayden, W.G., et al.: Radioisotopic angiocardiography: Findings in congenital heart disease. *J Nucl Med* 13:31-40, 1972.

5. Folse, R., and Braunwald, E.: Pulmonary vascular dilution curves recorded by external detection in the diagnosis of left-to-right shunts. *Br Heart J* 24:166-172, 1962.

6. Alazraki, N.P., Ashburn, W.L., Hagan, A., et al.: Detection of left-to-right cardiac shunts with the scintillation camera pulmonary dilution curve. *J Nucl Med* 13:142-147, 1972.

7. Hagan, A.D., Friedman, W.F., Ashburn, W.L., et al.: Further applications of scintillation scanning techniques to the diagnosis and management of infants and children with congenital heart disease. *Circulation* 45:858-868, 1972.

8. Rosenthall, L.: Qualitative and quantitative analysis of radionuclide cardiopulmonary histograms. *CRC Critical Reviews in Radiol Nuc Med* 5:479-493, 1974.

9. Rosenthall, L., and Mercer, E.N.: Intravenous radionuclide cardiography for the detection of cardiovascular shunts. *Radiology* 106:601-606, 1973.

10. Anderson, P.A.W., Jones, R.H., and Sabiston, D.C.: Quantitation of left-to-right cardiac shunts with radionuclide angiography. *Circulation* 49:512-516, 1974.

11. Maltz, D.L., and Treves, S.: Quantitative radionuclide angiocardiography: Determination of Qp:Qs in children. *Circulation* 47:1049-1056, 1973.

12. Alderson, P.O., Jost, R.G., Strauss, H.W., et al.: Radionuclide angiocardiography: Improved diagnosis and quantitation of left-to-right shunts using area ratio techniques in children. *Circulation* 51:1136-1143, 1975.

13. Alderson, P.O., Gaudiana, V.A., Watson, D.C., et al.: Quantitative radionuclide angiocardiography in animals with experimental atrial septal defects. *J Nucl Med* 19:364-369, 1978.

14. Askenazi, J., Ahnberg, D.S., Korngold, E., et al.: Quantitative radionuclide angiocardiography: Detection and quantitation of left-to-right shunts. *Am J Card* 37:382-278, 1976.

15. Strauss, H.W., Hurley, P.J., Rhodes, B.A., et al.: Quantification of right-to-left transpulmonary shunts in man. *J Lab Clin Med* 74:597-606, 1969.

16. Gates, G.F., Orme, H.W., and Dore, E.K.: Measurement of cardiac shunting with technetium-labeled albumin aggregates. *J Nucl Med* 12:746-749, 1971.

17. Hine, G.J., and Johnston, R.E.: Absorbed dose from radionuclides. *J Nucl Med* **11**:468, 1970.
18. Kurtz, D., Ahnberg, D.S., Freed, M., et al.: Quantitative radionuclide angiocardiography. Determination of left ventricular ejection fraction in children. *Br Heart J* **38**:966-973, 1976.
19. Burow, R.D., Strauss, H.W., Singleton, R., et al.: Analysis of left ventricular function from multiple gated acquisition cardiac blood pool imaging. *Circulation* **56**:1024-1028, 1977.
20. Marshall, R.C., Berger, H.J., Costin, J.C., et al.: Assessment of cardiac performance with quantitative radionuclide angiocardiography: Sequential left ventricular ejection fraction, normalized left ventricular ejection fraction rate, and regional wall motion. *Circulation* **56**:820-829, 1977.
21. Steele, P., Kirch, D., Matthews, M., et al. Measurement of left heart ejection fraction and end-diastolic volume by a computerized, scintigraphic technique using a wedged pulmonary arterial catheter. *Am J Card* **34**:179-186, 1974.
22. Hecht, H.S., Mirell, S.G., Rolett, E.L., et al.: Left-ventricular ejection fraction and segmental wall motion by peripheral first-pass radionuclide angiography. *J Nucl Med* **19**:17-23, 1978.
23. Jengo, J.A., Mena, I., Blaufuss, A., et al.: Evaluation of left ventricular function (ejection fraction and segmental wall motion) by single pass radioisotope angiography. *Circulation* **57**:326-332, 1978.
24. Reichek, N., Shelburne, J.C., and Perloff, J.K.: Clinical aspects of rheumatic valvular disease. *Prog Cardiovasc Dis* **15**:491-537, 1973.
25. Rigo, P., Alderson, P.O., Robertson, R.M., et al.: Measurement of aortic and mitral regurgitation by gated cardiac blood pool scans. *Circulation*, submitted for publication.
26. Strauss, H.W., Pitt, B., Rouleau, J., et al.: Congenital heart disease. In *Atlas of Cardiovascular Nuclear Medicine* C.V. Mosby, St. Louis, 1977, pp. 176-182.

CHAPTER XVIII

Radionuclide Evaluation of Peripheral Venous Disease

Ramesh C. Verma, M.D.

Since Virchow's first description of venous thrombosis, the incidence of this disease has been steadily rising.[1] It has been conservatively estimated in the past that venous thromboembolism causes 50,000 deaths anually in the United States.[2] The most serious complication of thrombophlebitis is pulmonary embolism, and up to 41 percent of patients with deep vein thrombosis of the lower extremity can develop pulmonary embolism.[3] Deep vein thrombosis is diagnosed before death in only 50 percent of all patients with fatal pulmonary emboli.[4] Deep vein thrombosis is present in the lower extremities in 67 percent of all patients in whom pulmonary embolism has been documented.[3] The classical clinical criteria for diagnosis of thrombophlebitis have been shown by various authors to have poor sensitivity.[5] This unreliability of the clinical signs has led to the development of a number of improved diagnostic methods. The newer techniques have allowed better estimates of the incidence of venous thrombosis in the high risk population; they have provided increased understanding of natural history of the disease; and they have determined the efficacy of certain therapeutic regimens for prevention and treatment of thrombophlebitis.

Radiographic venography is probably the oldest technique for confirmation of deep vein thrombosis. It is regarded as the "gold standard" against which newer tests for thrombosis detection are compared. Briefly, iodinated contrast medium is injected into one of the superficial pedal veins. Roentgenograms show the progress of the contrast solution through the veins. Tourniquets above the ankle and knee are generally applied to direct flow through the deep veins. A persistent filling defect (partial or complete) in the column of contrast medium in the vein suggests thrombus. When a vein is occluded, the collateral venous vessels fill with contrast solution. Free-floating thrombi are diagnosed by translucent area within the lumen of a vein with a rim of contrast around it.

The accuracy of radiographic venography varies, but it is generally believed that 90 percent to 95 percent of all thrombi may be detected in advanced radiographic laboratories. Smaller thrombi, including early stages of endothelial damage, may be missed. Not only does a radiographic venogram confirm the presence of a thrombus, it also defines its extent and, occasionally, the age (by degree of fixation to the vein wall) of the thrombus. This procedure also provides detailed information of other defects in the venous system. The disadvantages of radiographic venography include discomfort to the patient, contrast dye reactions, and occasionally phlebitis. The latter may necessitate temporary hospitalization. In patients with swollen feet, it is sometimes difficult to find a vein to inject the large amount of contrast medium. Moreover, venography is an invasive technique and has to be performed by highly trained personnel. In addition, patients must be moved from the ward. Hence, it is unsuitable for mass screening or for following the course of the disease with serial studies.

Over the past few years, a number of nuclear medical techniques for detection of thrombophlebitis have come of age. These include:
1. radionuclide venography (RNV) or isotope venography which usually consists of:
   a. flow study, and
   b. static or "hot spot" scan
2. fibrinogen uptake test (FUT)
3. newer procedures including scans following administration of radio-labelled fibrinogen or platelets.

Radionuclide Venography

As mentioned earlier, radionuclide venography is a two-part test. The first part, an isotope venogram, involves imaging of flow through the veins while a radio-tracer is injected into the veins of the foot. The second part, also referred to as the "hot spot" or the delayed scan, involves static imaging of legs soon after the flow study is completed. The "hot spot" scan detects regions of abnormal retention of tracer, especially in areas of endothelial damage of partially occluding thrombi.

Principle

The flow study, first used by Rosenthal et al.,[6] is based on the fact that when small quantities of tracer are introduced into the deep veins of the foot, the tracer is uniformly mixed in the blood and flows through the deep veins of the leg. Hence, where there is an area of total obstruction, a break will be demonstrated in the column of "radioactive blood". Collateral channels may be visualized, and these are indirect indications of obstruction. The "hot spot" scan, first developed by Webber et al.[7] in 1969, exploits the physical affinity between damaged endothelium (with the associated deposit of fibrin) and macroaggregates of albumin (MAA). The radiolabelled particles adhere to sites of damaged endothelium and partially occluded thrombi when they flow through these areas.

Test Procedure

The technique for isotope venography is similar to that used for radiographic venography. The only significant difference is that the amount of radiopharmaceutical injected is small (3 to 5 cc versus 100 cc of iodinated dye used for radiographic venography) and, unlike the contrast medium, the radiopharmaceuticals have no known effects on the venous endothelium. Many radiopharmaceuticals can be used to visualize venous flow, but the common ones are ^{99m}Tc-labelled MAA or microspheres of albumin or ^{99m}Tc-sulfur colloid. If a delayed or "hot spot" scan and a perfusion lung scan are to be obtained, the ^{99m}Tc-labelled MAA or microspheres are the agents of choice.

Tourniquets are applied above the patient's ankles and knees. In patients with varicose veins, firm wrapping of the legs with elastic bandages aids in preventing blood flow through the superficial veins of the lower extremity. A single injection or, often, a series of injections of radio-tracer are made through dorsal pedal veins, and a series of scans of the legs and pelvis are taken. The scintillation camera is moved along the length of the legs, or the patient is placed on a table which moves past a large field of view gamma camera. After the flow through the venous system has been defined, the legs are exercised, the tourniquets removed, and delayed static images are taken of the legs and pelvis. These delayed images detect retention of radio-particles at sites of thrombosis. If labelled MAA or microspheres are used for radionuclide venography, pulmonary perfusion scintigraphy may be done without administering any additional radiopharmaceutical.

Interpretation

Knowledge of the venous anatomy of legs and pelvis is essential for accurate interpretation of radionuclide venography (Fig. 18-1). With the application of tourniquets, no detectable flow is visualized through the superficial system in a normal individual. However, when tourniquets

VEINS OF LOWER LIMB

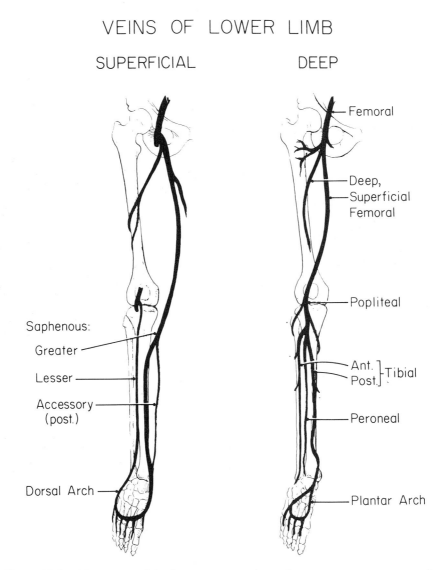

Figure 18-1. Major veins of the lower extremity (semi-diagrammatic representation).

are not used, flow may be seen in the deep veins in addition to the superficial veins. The normal static study (Fig. 18-2) reveals minimal

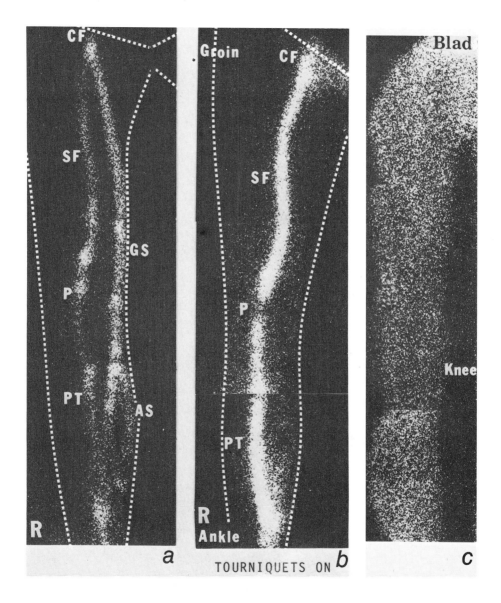

Figure 18-2. *A* and *B*, Venous channels of the right lower extremity commonly demonstrated in the anterior projection by nuclear venography. Superficial: Accessory Saphenous (AS) and Greater Saphenous (GS). Deep: Posterior Tibial (PT), Popliteal (P), Superficial Femoral (SF), Common Femoral (CF). The dotted lines represent the outlines of the extremity. *C*, Normal delayed static "hot spot" scan. Urinary bladder (Blad).

diffuse radioactivity along the entire leg and pelvis. However, in patients with thrombophlebitis, the radionuclide accumulates in "hot spots" (Fig. 18-3, A and B) which persist even after the leg has been exercised. The

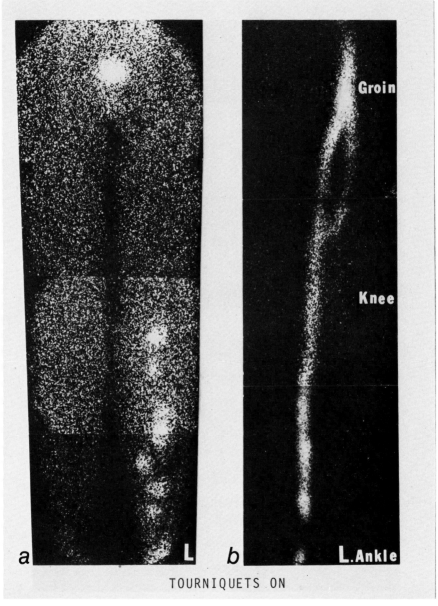

TOURNIQUETS ON

Figure 18-3.   *A* and *B*, Delayed static scan showing multiple "hot spots" in the left calf and knee regions with an isotope venogram of the same leg demonstrating absence of flow through the deep veins of the calf and popliteal region. Most of the flow in the latter areas occurs through the superficial greater saphenous vein.

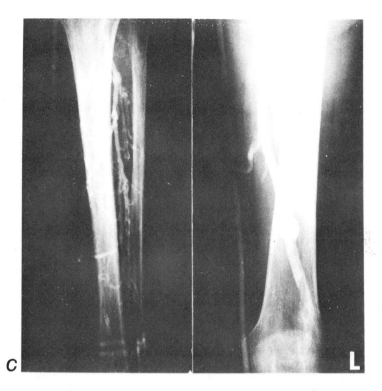

Figure 18-3.C, Radiographic contrast venogram on the same leg confirms the presence of thrombi in deep veins of calf and popliteal veins.

vigorous exercise helps exclude radioparticles trapped in static pools of blood, especially underneath valve cusps. Areas of minimal retention of radiolabelled particles below the knee may occur in approximately 20 percent of normal individuals.[8] Nuclear venograms provide an indirect method of diagnosis, based upon demonstration of absent or markedly-diminished venous flow, with or without associated flow through venous collaterals. The exact cause of venous occlusion cannot be made on the basis of nuclear venography alone. An extrinsic hematoma may cause narrowing of the venous lumen without obvious intraluminal thrombosis. However, if this narrowing is associated with a "hot spot" on the delayed scan, the diagnosis of thrombophlebitis is more definitive. Some veins show localized focal defects while their proximal and distal portions are well visualized. Such images must be interpreted with caution, since these defects may be the result of dilution by "nonradioactive blood" from the tributaries. A focal area of diminished flow in the popliteal vein may represent a normal variant.[9]

An example of a patient with an abnormal flow through the deep veins of the left calf and left popliteal vein and abnormal "hot spots" in the corresponding areas on the static scan is shown in Figure 18-3, A, B and C. A more detailed discussion of technique and interpretation of radio-nuclide venograms is available in the literature.[9,10]

Accuracy

The correlation of findings in radiographic and isotopic venography and the "hot spot" scan can be better understood by referring to the diagram in Figure 18-4. This diagramatic sketch represents a vein with an area of endothelial damage, a partially-occluding thrombus, and, higher up, an occlusive thrombus. Because of this occlusion, the venous flow has been directed through a collateral channel. A radiographic venogram (contrast phlebogram) will demonstrate the filling defects

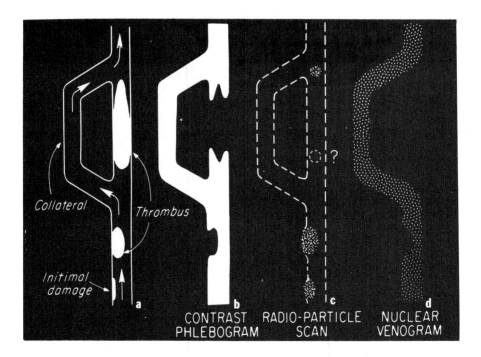

Figure 18-4. Diagrammatic representation of the three major steps (intimal damage, partially occlusive, and occlusive) of a thrombus (*a*) and the corresponding findings on a radiographic venogram (*b*), a "hot spot" scan (*c*), and a nuclear venogram (*d*) are shown. (For detailed explanation, please see text).

caused by the partially-occluding and occlusive thrombus and also the collateral channel. However, intimal damage may not be visualized. The nuclear venogram (Fig. 18-4D) will demonstrate narrowing (or diminished flow) through the region of the partially-occluding thrombus and will demonstrate an absence of flow in the region of totally-occluding thrombus, as well as flow along the collateral channel. A nuclear venogram will, however, miss sites of endothelial damage or small thrombi. A delayed scan or the radio-particle scan (Fig. 18-4C), on the other hand, will demonstrate "hot spots" in regions where the radio-particles come in contact with the damaged endothelium and partially-occluding thrombi. It may miss occlusive thrombi completely, depending upon how much of the occlusive thrombus is in the path of flow of blood through the collateral channels. In summary then, a site-by-site correlation between radiographic and nuclear venogram or "hot spot" scans does not always exist. A "hot spot" scan may miss all total occlusions, and an isotope venogram (flow study) may miss all areas of early endothelial damage and small thrombi. Combination of the two parts of the radionuclide venogram will, however, allow detection of over 90 percent of all radiographically-demonstrated thrombi.[9,11] The false positive rate is higher for delayed static scans because they demonstrate endothelial lesions generally not shown on contrast phlebography.

This chapter deals primarily with the use of RNV in the lower extremities and the pelvis. There are, however, other important applications of RNV which include (a) confirmation of thrombophlebitis in the upper extremities, (b) documentation of obstruction (extrinsic or intrinsic) in the subclavian veins, e.g., in thoracic outlet syndromes, and (c) evaluation of superior vena cava obstruction in patients with mediastinal masses.

Risks and Complications

Radionuclide venography, like most other nuclear medicine procedures, is considered a noninvasive procedure. The risks are those associated with the venipuncture and the injected radiopharmaceutical. To prevent infection, strict aseptic techniques must be followed, especially in patients with swollen feet. The estimated absorbed radiation dose from 4 millicuries of ^{99m}Tc-MAA to the target organ, the lungs, is less than 200 millirads. Unlike the radiographic contrast venogram, no evidence of worsening of a patient's symptoms has been reported following a radionuclide venogram.

Fibrinogen Uptake Test

Palko and his associates first reported use of radiolabelled fibrinogen in detection of thrombi in patients.[12] However, the clinical value of I-125 labelled fibrinogen was not realized until 1968 when Flanc, Kakkar, and Clarke[14] and, independently, Negus and his associates[15] confirmed the results of I-125 fibrinogen studies for detection of deep vein thrombosis (DVT) with contrast phlebography. The test was subsequently simplified by Kakkar et al., so that it can now be performed at the patient's bedside.[16]

Principle

When homologous fibrinogen is labelled with radioactive iodine and injected, it behaves like the patient's own fibrinogen. If administered before or while a thrombus is formed, radioactive fibrinogen is incorporated into the active thrombus. The amount of radionuclide incorporated in the forming thrombus is generally higher than in the circulating blood and the associated inflammatory reaction is greater in the thrombus than in the muscle background. Hence, radionuclide counts will be higher in regions of thrombosis.

Test Procedure

The procedure involves administering I-125 labelled fibrinogen intravenously after the thyroid gland has been blocked with oral Lugol's iodine or saturated solution of potassium iodide. The I-125 counts over the cardiac blood pool and at several marked sites (along the path of major veins in the lower extremity) are obtained daily for a week. High risk patients may be given I-125 fibrinogen and then monitored for one or two weeks or until the test becomes positive. The radioisotope counts measured in the leg are expressed as a percentage of the cardiac blood pool counts.

Interpretation

The results of the counts measured in the leg can be tabulated (Table 18-1) or plotted on a graph for easier interpretation (Fig. 18-5). In normal studies, the percent reading decreased gradually from the inguinal ligament down to the ankle, often with slight increase over the knees. In a normal individual, these readings do not increase on subsequent days. A study is interpreted as abnormal if a significant increase

TABLE 18-1
Count Ratio of Precordial to Leg Radioactivity

Leg	Right		Left	
Positions	Day 1	Day 2	Day 1	Day 2
Groin				
1	55	50	53	50
2	52	46	48	43
3	40	37	38	41
4	37	37	39	36
5	35	38	36	31
Knee				
1	36	38	40	34
2	35	37	44	42
3	33	32	57	64
4	31	30	58	60
5	29	25	40	36
Ankle				

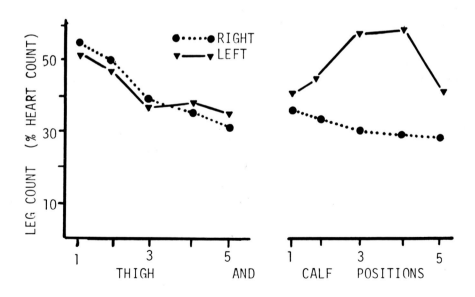

Figure 18-5. Fibrinogen Uptake Test (FUT): Graphic representation of test results for right and left legs for day 1 only from Table 18-1. The left leg is normal. The uptake in the right lower calf demonstrates a significant abnormal increase in counts.

in counts, persistent over 24 hours, is observed at any of the marked sites on the leg. This significant increase is determined by comparing corresponding sites on the contralateral leg, adjacent sites on the same leg, or the same site on two different days. A "significant" rise may amount to 15 percent or 20 percent points (all values being expressed as a ratio of precordial to leg activity × 100). This test is positive in two-thirds of the patients with existing thrombophlebitis in three to four hours after the I-125 fibrinogen was injected and in most others, 24 hours after injection.[17]

Accuracy

The sensitivity of the fibrinogen uptake test in diagnosis of deep vein thrombosis is over 90 percent. The specificity of the test depends on the type of patients included in the study. However, if potential false-positive lesions, that is, those that are known to have increased deposit of I-125 fibrinogen (cellulitis, abscess, hematoma, ulcers, arthritis, fractures, and gross edema) are excluded, the specificity is also in the range of 90 percent. The greatest strength of the fibrinogen uptake test lies in its ability to demonstrate forming thrombi. It is generally believed that the fibrinogen uptake test yields positive results so long as the fibrinogen is being deposited into the area of the thrombus and may be positive for up to four days following anticoagulation. The test is less likely to be positive in fully-formed or old thrombi. This is a distinct advantage over the radionuclide venogram and the contrast phlebogram which cannot always differentiate between new and old thrombi. The greatest limitation of the fibrinogen uptake test is that it takes at least 24 hours before the results can be interpreted definitively. Many factors compromise the sensitivity of the fibrinogen uptake test for detecting thrombi above the mid thigh. One of the factors is the high background counts in the upper thigh caused by radioactivity in the vessels or by scattered counts from the I-125 excreted in the urinary bladder. In addition, the low energy of Iodine-125 causes attenuation of gamma ray emissions and, hence, loss of counts from deep-seated veins. For the same reasons, the fibrinogen uptake test has essentially no role in detection of thrombi in the pelvic veins. The FUT lends itself well to serial studies for up to ten days after a single intravenous injection of the tracer. An added advantage is that the entire procedure can be performed at the patient's bedside by using a portable counting device. While it is a simple test to perform, the procedure itself and the calculation following the actual counting are time-consuming. Since fibrinogen is known to be deposited during all healing processes in the body, the test can yield false-positive results at sites of inflammation listed earlier. Homologous fibrinogen, which has previously been screened for hepatitis- associated antigen, has been used extensively in Europe for the fibrinogen uptake test without any evidence of hepatitis attributible to the Iodine-125 fibrinogen. I-125 fibrinogen is currently available commercially in the United States for routine use.

Risks and Complications

Fibrinogen uptake test is essentially noninvasive. The risks of complications following venipuncture are even less than those associated with RNV, since I-125 fibrinogen can be injected through any vein in the body. The usual amount of fibrinogen injected is less than 1 mg. The fibrinogen used is obtained by repeated plasmapheresis of a small number of carefully screened donors. The recipients of fibrinogen prepared from such carefully selected donors must also be followed for at least six months to insure that infusion of such material does not cause transmission of clinical or subclinical hepatitis, as demonstrated by hepatitis-associated antigen (HAA) or induction of an HAA antibody response in these recipients. In one large reported series[9] from England, no evidence of clinical hepatitis has been discovered in over 2,500 patients studied.

The amount of radiation exposure to the target organ, blood, from 100 microcuries of I-125 fibrinogen is 200 millirads.

Newer Isotopic Procedures

Fibrinogen Scans

Iodine-131[18] and Iodine-123[19] labelled fibrinogen have been used for imaging thrombi in lower extremities. The greatest advantage of these radionuclides over radioactive fibrinogen is that images rather than counts are taken. Moreover, unlike the fibrinogen uptake test (FUT), the fibrinogen scans can identify thrombi in the upper thigh and pelvis. Compared to the fibrinogen uptake test, the I-123 fibrinogen scan also has better spatial resolution because of the more suitable imaging characteristics of I-123 for gamma scintillation cameras. The lesions are generally better visualized on the delayed (24 hours post-injection) images because of diminution in the blood background. However, because of the short physical half-life of I-123 (13.3 hours), delayed scans are not very practical. Neither I-131 nor I-123 labelled fibrinogen are commercially available for routine use. Experience with these agents is currently limited, and further trials are needed to determine their role.

Radiolabelled Platelets

Autologous platelets have been labelled with Indium-111 oxine and shown, both in experimental animals[20] and man,[21] to accumulate in sites of endothelial damage and thrombophlebitis. The labelling techniques have not been perfected, and hence preliminary results from various centers are inconsistent. The advantages of Indium-111 platelet scans would be that the physical characteristics of Indium-111 are better than I-123 fibrinogen. Further clinical trials are needed to establish the practicality and efficacy of In-111 platelet scintigraphy for diagnosis of deep vein thrombosis.

Optimal Use of Radionuclide Procedures

The nuclear venogram is most helpful in demonstrating total occlusions and collateral vessels, both of which are strong indicators of venous thrombosis. The delayed "hot spot" scan is a good technique for evaluating early intimal damage and partially occlusive thrombi. The delayed scan may, however, miss total occlusions, hence the importance of combining it with the flow study to detect all stages of thrombophlebitis. Radionuclide venography can demonstrate abnormalities in pelvic veins. However, radionuclide venography cannot differentiate old from new disease. The test takes 30 to 45 minutes to complete. The results, which are available soon after completion of the test, are in a pictorial format (images) and, hence, easier to interpret.

In summary, radionuclide venography, therefore, is the test of choice (Table 18-2) for all patients suspected of having pelvic vein thrombi. Since the results of radionuclide venography are available within 30 to 45 minutes, it is an ideal technique for confirming deep vein thrombosis in patients with clinical signs suggesting this diagnosis, especially when an early diagnosis is desired to avoid unnecessary hospitalization and anticoagulation. Since most emboli to lungs originate from the iliofemoral veins, and since radionuclide venography is sensitive in these regions, it is recommended for all retrospective studies to document the source of a known pulmonary embolus. In patients who are sensitive to iodinated contrast media, radionuclide venography offers the only noninvasive alternative for demonstrating venous flow, although it lacks the fine anatomic definition of the radiographic venogram.

TABLE 18-2
Radionuclides Used to Detect Thrombosis

Radionuclide Venography: Test of choice for:
1. All patients suspected of having pelvic vein thrombi.
2. Confirmation of doubtful clinical diagnosis.
3. Documentation of origin of a pulmonary embolus.
4. Patients sensitive to iodinated contrast medium.

Fibrinogen Uptake Test: Test of choice for:
1. Prospective detection of venous thrombosis in high risk groups (e.g., acute myocardial infarction, post-operative states).
2. Evaluation for recurrence versus post-phlebitic syndrome in patients with documented history of deep vein thrombosis in the legs.
3. Unsuccessful venipuncture in patients with swollen ankles and feet.

The greatest strength of the fibrinogen uptake test lies in its ability to detect forming thrombi. However, the test has limited value in detecting thrombi in the upper thigh and pelvis. It takes at least 24 hours before a reliable interpretation of the results can be made. Serial studies can be performed conveniently up to seven days after a single injection of I-125 fibrinogen. The fibrinogen uptake test is also ideally suited for bedside examination, and therefore, should be the first test of choice (Table 18-2) when high risk individuals must be examined for thrombophlebitis, e.g., following surgery or myocardial infarction. Serial studies may be preferred for up to ten days, and appropriate treatment can be initiated early and as soon as the fibrinogen uptake test suggests presence of thrombophlebitis. This test is also the test of choice in patients with suspected recurrence of deep vein thrombosis, since radionuclide venography is not very helpful in differentiating old from new disease.

References

1. Ruckley, C.V.:   Venous thrombo-embolic disease.   *J Roy Coll Surg Edinb* **20**:10-24, 1975.
2. Wessler, S.:   A heparin symposium: Introduction. *Curr Ther Res* **18**:3-5, 1975.
3. Nelp, W.B.:   Radionuclide venography (RNV) in the practice of nuclear

medicine. *J Nucl Med* **18**:611, 1977.

4. Sevitt, S., and Gallagher, N.:   Venous thrombosis and pulmonary embolism: A clinico-pathological study in injured and burned patients. *Brit J Surg* **48**:475-489, 1961.

5. Johnson, W.C.:   Evaluation of new techniques for the diagnosis of venous thrombosis. *J Surg Res* **16**:473-481, 1974.

6. Rosenthall, L.:   Combined inferior venacavography, iliac venography and lung imaging with Tc99m albumin macroaggregates. *Radiology* **98**:623-626, 1971.

7. Webber, M.M., Bennett, L.R., Cragin, M., et al.:   Thrombophlebitis demonstration by scintiscanning. *Radiology* **92**:620-623, 1969.

8. Webber, M.M., Pollak, E.W., Victery, W., et al.:   Thrombosis detection by radionuclide particle (MAA) entrapment: Correlation with fibrinogen uptake and venography. *Radiology* **111**:645-650, 1974.

9. Verma, R.C., Webber, M.M., Ramanna, L.R., et al.:   Radionuclide venography and the role of radionuclides in the detection of venous disease. *Vasc Surg* **11**:227-240, 1977.

10. Hayt, D.B., Blatt, C.J., and Freeman, L.M.:   Radionuclide venography: Its place as a modality for the investigation of thromboembolic phenomena. *Sem Nucl Med* **7**:263-281, 1977.

11. Ennis, J.T., and Elmes, R.J.:   Radionuclide venography in the diagnosis of deep vein thrombosis. *Radiology* **125**:441-449, 1977.

12. Palko, P.D., Nanson, E.M., and Fedoruk, S.O.:   The early detection of deep vein thrombosis using I-131-tagged human fibrinogen. *Canad J Surg* **7**:215-226, 1964.

13. Kakkar, V.V.:   Fibrinogen uptake test for detection of deep vein thrombosis—A review of current practice. *Sem Nucl Med* **7**:229-244, 1977.

14. Flanc, C., Kakkar, V.V., and Clarke, M.B.:   The detection of venous thrombosis of the legs using I-125 fibrinogen. *Brit J Surg* **55**:742-747, 1968.

15. Negus, D., Pinto, D.L., LeQuesne, L.P., et al.:   I-125 labelled fibrinogen in the diagnosis of deep vein thrombosis and its correlation with phlebography. *Brit J Surg* **55**:835-839, 1968.

16. Kakkar, V.V., Nicolaides, A.N., Renney, J.T.G., et al.:   I-125 labelled fibrinogen test adapted for routine screening for deep vein thrombosis. *Lancet* **1**: 540-542, 1970.

17. DeNardo, G.L., DeNardo, S.J., Barnett, C.A., et al.:   Assessment of conventional criteria for the early diagnosis of thrombophlebitis with I-125 fibrinogen uptake test. *Radiology* **125**:765-768, 1977.

18. Charkes, N.D., Dugan, M.A., Maier, W.P., et al.:   Scintigraphic detection of deep-vein thrombosis with I-131 fibrinogen. *J Nucl Med* **15**:1163-1166, 1974.

19. DeNardo, S.J., and DeNardo, G.L.:   I-123 fibrinogen scintigraphy. *Sem Nucl Med* **7**:245-251, 1977.

20. Thakur, M.L., Welch, M.J., Joist, J.H., et al.: Indium-111 labelled platelets: Studies on preparation and evaluation of in vitro and in vivo functions. *Thromb Res* **9**:345-357, 1976.

21. Goodwin, D.A., Bushberg, J.T., Doherty, P.W., et al.: Indium-111 labelled autologous platelets for location of vascular thrombi in humans. *J Nucl Med* **19**:626-634, 1978.

CHAPTER XIX

Arterial Disease of the Lower Extremities

Michael E. Siegel, M.D., and
Charles A. Stewart, M.D.

The use of radioactive tracers in the evaluation of the patient with peripheral arterial disease has offered clinically useful information. Radionuclide studies can be used to: (1) detect small vessel disease by demonstrating regional perfusion in the microcirculation under various stresses; (2) determine patency of the vascular graft; (3) determine relative perfusion of "ischemic" ulcers and predict their healing potential; (4) detect and estimate size of arteriovenous shunts; and (5) evaluate potential for healing in surgical amputations by determining skin perfusion pressure.

Determination of Blood Flow

The clearance of highly diffusable tracers, deposited in the tissue of interest can be used to make objective measurements of blood flow. The local clearance method uses tracers that diffuse freely between the tissue and the capillary blood so that diffusion is maintained almost at equilibrium regardless of the rate of blood flow. When these tracers are used, the blood flow is the limiting factor in their removal from a locally injected depot. Radioactive xenon-133 is one such blood flow-limited tracer. After the tracer is deposited in the tissue an estimate of blood flow in milliliters/100 grams/minute (ml/100 gm/min) can be derived from the clearance rate of the tracer.[1]

Clearance rates in normals increase significantly with exercise. However, increased rate of clearance is also seen in patients with arterial vascular disease, in spite of intermittent claudication during the exercise. This supports the hypothesis that patients with symptomatic arterial vascular disease can increase blood flow to the symptomatic portion, but the relative increase may not be adequate to meet the increased demands. Clearance of ^{133}Xe is similar in normal individuals regardless of whether the examination is done during exercise or the procedures causing reactive hyperemia are used. The maximum clearance rate (peak reactive hyperemia) occurs within one minute after relief of the arterial occlusion. The maximum blood flow in ml/100 gm/min and the time until maximum blood flow is reached after release of the arterial occlusion is an estimate of the extent of involvement of the major arteries of the leg and, to some extent, the functioning of the collateral vessels. The patients with peripheral vascular disease have a delayed, diminished and prolonged response to the reactive hyperemia. With reactive hyperemia, maximum blood flow in patients with peripheral vascular disease is approximately 17 ml/100 gm/min while in normals under the same conditions, it is approximately 50 ml/100 gm/min. The figure widely accepted as representing resting blood flow in the normal individual is 20ml/100 gm/min. To be considered normal, the maximum flow should be reached within one minute after release of the occlusion pressure that induced the reactive hyperemia. Although the test has been reported to be sensitive (95 percent positive in patients with vascular disease between the heart and the site of measurement), false negative results are encountered in patients with good collateral circulation and in those which the lesion is close to the site of measurement.

An intramuscular injection of 0.1ml of sterile saline containing 0.5 μCi of ^{133}Xe has proven useful for this approach. A 27-gauge needle is inserted approximately one to two centimeters deep and the needle is left in place for approximately 30 seconds after completion of the injection. The injection is usually made in the anterior tibialis muscles about 10 cm inferior to the patella although some investigators inject into the gastrocnemius muscle. The appropriately collimated probe is placed ten cm from the skin, and constant geometry must be maintained during the procedure. Precautions are necessary to avoid injecting gas. (The gas: tissue partition coefficient for ^{133}Xe or ^{85}Kr is 10:1). The interpretation must, of course, take into account the cardiac status and metabolic state of the patient, for these too are reflected in the clearance data.

The flow rates are calculated by plotting on semi-log paper the activity versus time data which have been accumulated. The initial component is monoexponential. The half period (T½) is derived from the curve and from the following:

$$F = 100 \times \lambda \times \frac{0.693}{T½} \quad \text{where}$$

F equals cc/100 gm/min, and λ is the partition coefficient for the tissue being studied. Clearance half-time (T½) is then used to calculate blood flow in the area injected.

An additional application of the diffusible gas clearance approach is in the quantification of blood flow to the skin. Of particular interest was Serjrsen's findings of low flow values in the skin, particularly during and after exercise, in patients with peripheral vascular disease.[2] This finding was qualitatively verified by the peripheral perfusion scanning with and without reactive hyperemia, as reported by Siegel.[3] They found a relative decrease, during reactive hyperemia, of nonmuscular to muscular flow in many of the patients with peripheral vascular disease.

Lassen and others have used the skin perfusion pressures as measured by the ^{133}Xe washout approach to predict the healing ability of amputation stumps. They used ^{131}I or ^{125}I iodo-antipyrene rather than ^{133}Xe because xenon's high solubility causes it to diffuse into the subcutaneous fatty tissue. The iodo-antipyrene, 0.1 ml, is injected intradermally and counter-pressure is applied with a blood pressure cuff over the radioactive deposit. The skin perfusion pressure is that pressure at which washout and thus perfusion stops. In normal individuals, this pressure approximates diastolic pressure. In a study of skin perfusion pressure in 51 leg amputees, it was found that healing potential was greatest when the skin perfusion pressure was 40 mmHg or more.[1] The local clearance technique may also be used to determine the best level for amputation in patients with peripheral vascular disease. A procedure to amputate a lower extremity in the treatment of peripheral vascular disease, should combine maximum potential for rehabilitation with minimum morbidity and mortality. Despite improvement in surgical techniques for peripheral vascular disease, at present maximum rehabilitation with minimum morbidity remains a difficult goal to achieve. Not uncommonly, the surgeon must subject a patient to progressive levels of amputation and months of hospitalization before a viable, well-healed amputation stump can be obtained. A simplified approach taken by some is to select the level of amputation at the lowest level of skin viability as determined by testing for bleeding at the time of operation. The clinical test is nonspecific and does not take into consideration the ability of the skin to heal or to the degree of muscle ischemia. Of the many ancillary aids available to the surgeon, angiography is the most widely accepted. However, it provides only indirect inference to the actual perfusion of capillary beds, and most surgeons have become discouraged with this approach in determining the level of amputation. Perhaps somewhat more promising is the use of ^{133}Xe determined skin perfusion pressures, as previously described,[1] to determine the level at which healing will occur.

Lassen considers a pressure less than 20 to 30 mmHg unsatisfactory for healing and thus suggests considering of amputation at a better perfused proximal level.

Noninvasive Visualization of Major Vessels and Grafts

Isotope angiography performed noninvasively by the intravenous injection of ^{99m}Tc pertechnetate has proven to be a useful diagnostic tool in a variety of arterial disorders. Isotope angiography can be used to diagnose arterial stenosis, arterial occlusions, and true and false aneurysms.[4] It is useful as a screening technique in evaluating traumatic arterial injury and recently has been used postoperatively to assess arterial and graft patency.[5,6] It is especially useful in long-term follow-up of patients who have had surgery. Although it provides poorer anatomic resolution than conventional contrast angiography, with good technique, isotope angiography can accurately demonstrate the arterial system of the extremities to the level of the mid-calf and the wrist.[7]

This technique involves the use of a scintillation camera with a high resolution, low-energy all purpose collimator. The patient is positioned under the camera with the arterial area of interest centered in the field of view. Approximately 10 to 15 millicuries of ^{99m}Tc pertechnetate in a volume of 1 ml or less is injected as a bolus into an antecubital fossa vein. A good bolus injection is critical to the success of the procedure. Serial scintiphoto images are taken at 2 to 3 second intervals. Immediately following the dynamic portion of the study, a single 300,000 count static exposure is made; and if there is clincial suspicion of aneurysm or extravasation, another static image is taken after a delay of 10 to 15 minutes. Moss et al. have reported results of 253 isotope angiograms on a variety of patients with good clinical, surgical, or contrast angiographic correlation.[4] In normal subjects the abdominal aorta, common and external iliac, common superficial, and deep femoral, popliteal, axillary, brachial, radial, and ulnar arteries were well demonstrated. A rapid and unimpeded flow through the visualized artery could be interpreted as a sign that there was no significant intraluminal disease. Total vascular occlusions were also apparent. Stenotic lesions that appear greater than 30 percent occluded on contrast angiography could be visually detected as luminal narrowing on the isotope angiogram. Aneurysms were seen as a widened lumen representing the aneurysmal sac or as a narrowed, tortuous lumen surrounded by an area of almost no activity representing clot within the aneurysm. In cases of trauma, extraluminal accumulations of tracer represent acute hemorrhage or false aneurysm formation. These findings are usually apparent on the dynamic studies but may be demonstrated only on the delayed static images in some cases. Rudavsky et al.[5] have reported a group of patients with suspected traumatic arterial injuries who underwent isotope angiograms as a screening procedure and had 90 percent true positives and 90 percent true negatives as confirmed by contrast angiography. Thus isotope angiography has the potential of being a good noninvasive screening procedure for traumatic arterial injury and can aid in the selection of patients requiring contrast angiography.

Perhaps the most efficacious use of isotope angiography is the postoperative evaluation of the patency of surgical bypass grafts. In the postoperative period when the limb is swollen and obscured by dressing, assessment by palpation of pulses is difficult. It is also best to avoid arterial catheterization in those patients who have pre-existing arterial disease and are on anticoagulation therapy.[6] Moss et al. reported on a series of patients who had arterial reconstruction.[7] Early diagnosis in such cases is the key to successful healing. Isotope angiography is a more acceptable form of follow-up than contrast angiography in such cases, since it can be repeated frequently and is better tolerated by the patient because of its noninvasive nature.

Newer Noninvasive Techniques for Measuring Regional Blood Flow

Regional Blood Flow

Another approach which certainly warrants further investigation is the use of intravenously administered tracers such as ^{43}K or ^{201}Tl to visualize the distribution of perfusion in the extremities. As will be apparent in the following pages, the microsphere peripheral vascular perfusion study has yielded clinically useful information regarding the identification of physiologically significant vascular lesions, evaluating effectiveness of collateral circulation, and predicting ulcer healing potential of the skin. However, because of the particulate nature of the tracer, the microsphere perfusion study must be performed via an intra-arterial injection; and to compare perfusion in both lower extremities, the tracer must be delivered into the abdominal aorta.

Thallium-201 is a nonparticulate, monovalent, cation tracer. It has been demonstrated that the accumulation of thallium-201 in the heart is related to regional myocardial blood flow.[8] More recently, it has been shown that in skeletal muscle, thallium-201 distribution reflects the fractional distribution of cardiac output and is thus related to regional blood flow.[9] We have chosen to evaluate the efficacy of this tracer in the noninvasive evaluation of the distribution of blood flow perfusion at rest and during stress in the lower extremities.

The initial study reported on the qualitative and quantitative distribution of thallium-201 in the normal extremity.[10] As was noted in the microsphere studies, they found that: (1) The distribution of perfusion was primarily proportional to muscle mass with a relative hypoperfusion of nonmuscular structures such as knees and ankles. (2) The perfusion per unit area over the thigh can be as much as 50 percent greater than in the calf. (3) There is symmetry of perfusion between the extremities. (4) The calf-to-ankle perfusion increased an average of 91 percent with exercise. (5) The thigh to knee perfusion increased an average of 85 percent with exercise (Fig. 19-1). Initial studies with patients who have documented peripheral vascular disease suggest that thallium-201 extremity scans reveal similar distribution of radioactivity as seen after the microsphere injection (Fig. 19-2).

Regional Distribution of Blood Flow Using Radioactive Microspheres

Arteriography provides detailed anatomical information of the larger vessels, a necessity in the preoperative evaluation of the patient with peripheral vascular disease. However, the physiologic significance of the intravascular pathology and its ability to restrict perfusion to the regional capillary beds is not directly evaluated by what is, essentially, a morphologic technique. With reconstructive vascular surgery becoming more commonplace, defining the physiologic significance of a lesion should prove useful in patient selection and choice of operative approach. Moreover, many of these same patients are often burdened with ischemic ulcers, and the question of disfiguring surgery versus conservative therapy arises. An evaluation of the capillaries ability to perfuse the ulcer bed should provide a useful prognostic index. The particle distribution method for determining regional distribution of blood flow permits evaluation of the distribution of perfusion at the level of the microcirculation and the effect of intravascular pathology on this distribution.

The method was introduced clinically in 1964 for the determination of regional pulmonary perfusion and has since been applied to the heart, as well as to the extremities.[11]

It should be remembered, however, that the tracers do not yield, by themselves, direct quantitative data of blood flow but permit quan-

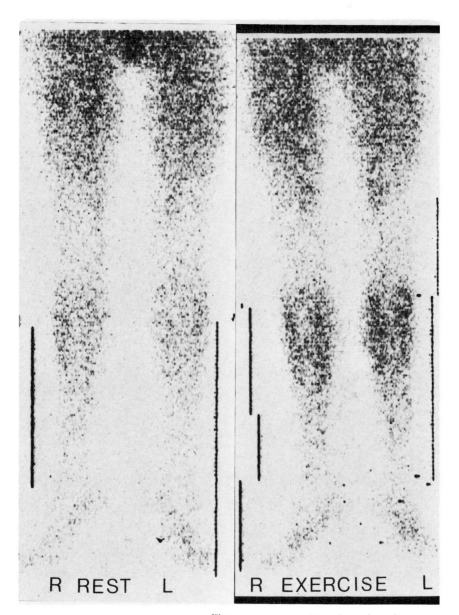

R REST L   R EXERCISE L

Figure 19-1. Normal distribution of ^{201}Tl in a 52-year-old male with no known peripheral vascular disease at rest (left) and during stress (right). Relative perfusion to muscular structures increases with stress.

tification only of the relative distribution of perfusion. Siegel reported on a large group of normal subjects and patients with peripheral vascular

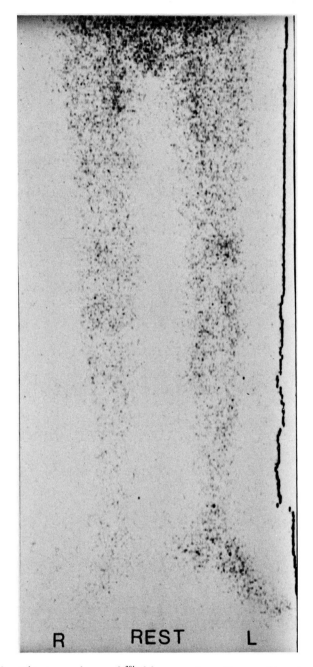

Figure 19-2. This is an abnormal ^{201}Tl leg scan in a 45-year-old male with juvenile diabetes, bilateral intermittent calf claudication, and a 60 percent narrowing of his right popliteal artery as the only lesion noted on angiography. Except for a slight relative hypoperfusion of the distal right extremity, there is a homogeneous distribution of the tracer.

disease studied by the particle distribution method. Injections of 5 to 10 millicuries of ^{99m}Tc-labeled albumin microspheres were injected either intra-aortically, via a translumbar approach, or via direct femoral artery catheterization with a Teflon-sheathed 19-gauge needle. The patients were then scanned anteriorly and posteriorly with a dual 5-inch scanner using 1:5 minification. The distribution of radioactivity in the extremity was categorized into five distinct peripheral perfusion patterns.[10]

The first of the patterns, seen in patients with no known peripheral vascular disease and identical to the pattern seen in normal thallium-201 scans, demonstrates the activity to be distributed in proportion to muscle mass with a relative decrease in radioactivity in the nonmuscular regions, i.e., the knees and the ankles. In the second pattern the activity is distributed more in proportion to skin surface rather than to muscle mass, with a more or less homogeneous distribution of activity (Fig. 19-3). This pattern is frequently seen in scans of patients with symptoms of ischemia, with essentially normal arteriograms, and scans of patients with diabetes. It is thought these patients have diffuse small vessel disease below the resolution of the arteriogram. The third pattern demonstrates an increase in the relative perfusion of the nonmuscular structures, i.e., knees and ankles, while the major muscle masses remain easily identifiable. This pattern is seen in patients with known multifocal disease of the large vessels. The fourth pattern demonstrates marked asymmetry in the distribution of radioactivity with a relative hypoperfusion of one or more of the muscle masses. This pattern, seen in patients with "ischemic" ulcers of the distal extremity, demonstrates increased activity in the ulcer bed (Fig. 19-4). The fifth pattern demonstrates increased activity in the osseous structures of the extremity. This pattern was seen in patients with Paget's disease of fibrous dysplasia involving the lower extremities.

One prerequisite for a new diagnostic or prognostic procedure to be accepted is that it should offer previously obtainable information more easily or offer new, potentially clinically useful information about a disease process. We conducted a study correlating the clinical, radioisotope scan, and arteriographic findings in a group of patients with symptomatic peripheral vascular disease. We found that the scan does not necessarily offer the same information as the other two modalities and, indeed, may offer useful physiologic information concerning the arterial pathology.[13] There was, as expected, a poor correlation between the radionuclide scans and the arteriograms, with 20 percent of patients demonstrating more and 40 percent less extensive disease on scans than on arteriograms. It was noted that the majority of the patients with extensive disease on the scan were diabetics who had essentially normal

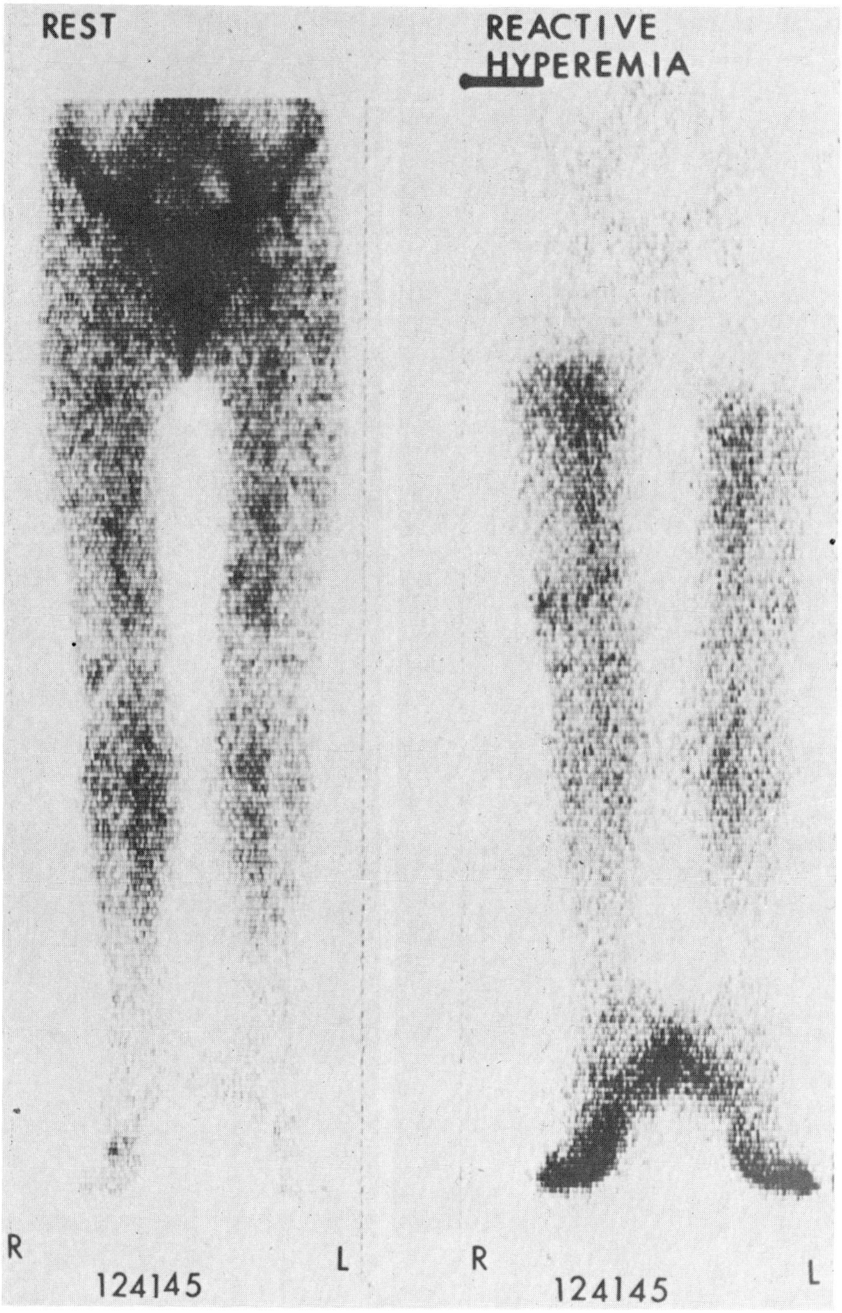

Figure 19-3.   Abnormal rest (left) and stress (right) microsphere perfusion study demonstrating diffuse small vessel disease pattern in a patient with claudication and a normal arteriorgram. (Reproduced with permission from Siegel, M.E., Giargiana, F.A., Rhodes, B.A., et al.: Effect of reactive hyperemia on the distribution of radioactive microspheres in patients with periphereal vascular disease. *Am J Roentgen* **118**:814, 1974).

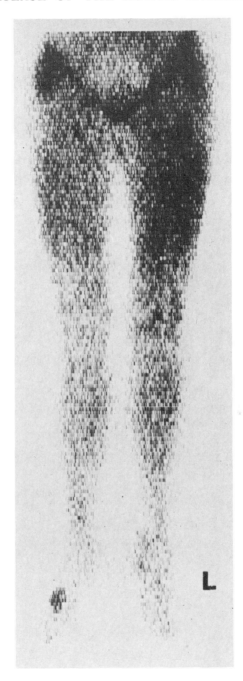

Figure 19-4. Relatively hyperperfused ulcer on the patient's right foot. (Reproduced with permission from Siegel, M.E., and Wagner, H.N., Jr.: Radioactive tracers in peripheral vascular disease. *Sem Nucl Med* **6**:253, 1976.)

REST

REACTIVE
HYPEREMIA

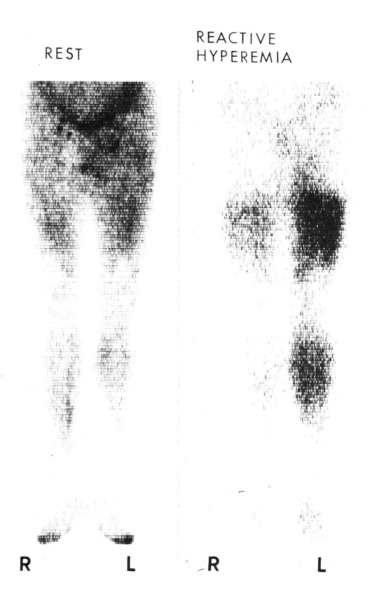

R   L   R   L

Figure 19-5. The differential response of the legs to stress is well demonstrated in the microsphere leg scan. The right side, especially the calf, responds less effectively to stress than does the left. (Reproduced with permission from Siegel, M.E., and Wagner, H.N., Jr.: Radioactive tracers in peripheral vascular disease. *Sem Nucl Med* **6**:253, 1976.)

arteriograms and scans which suggested diffuse small vessel disease. In fact, the scans were often the only objective evidence of diffuse arterial involvement in these patients. This is a particularly important point because establishing the presence of diffuse small vessel disease on the scan, even in the absence of significant disease of the angiogram, can aid the physician in avoiding an expensive, time-consuming work-up searching for a cause for the patient's symptoms.

One evaluation of regional perfusion that has already proven to be prognostically significant is the evaluation of "ischemic" ulcers. It is often difficult to determine whether a lesion will heal with conservative management or whether a disfiguring operation is necessary in these patients. Previous guidelines were often inadequate, leading to prolonged hospitalization or premature surgery. The term "ischemic ulcer" is used to denote a skin lesion with tissue loss as a result of arterial disease.

Inherent in the healing process is the tissue's ability to develop an inflammatory response and hyperemia which are necessary requirements for this revitalization process. As previously described, after intra-arterial injections of degradable radioactive human serum albumin microspheres (15 to 30 μ in diameter), the relative blood flow in the extremity is proportional to the distribution of microspheres, and this distribution can be visualized and quantitated by scintillation scanning. In patients with arterial disease, the arterioles may be maximally dilated as a result of ischemia, and no further response is possible in areas of injury or infection. Thus, the ratio of activity per unit area of lesion to that of neighboring healthy tissue reflects the degree of ischemia on a local or microcirculatory level, which in turn may predict whether or not the lesion will heal with conservative measures (Fig. 19-5).

Radioisotope Tracer Methods and Shunt Detection in the Extremities

One of the more elegant uses of radioactive microsphere studies has been in the detection of arteriovenous shunting in patients with Paget's disease or hypertrophic pulmonary osteoarthropathy. Radionuclide particles which are larger than the capillary diameter become trapped in the capillary bed in proportion to regional perfusion. However, if arteriovenous communication is present, these microspheres will travel to the lungs. Thus, quantitation of radioactivity over the lungs after injection of radioactive microspheres in a peripheral artery will reflect on the precapillary arteriovenous communication. Rhodes et al. using this technique evaluated patients with Paget's disease and demonstrated a lack of anatomic shunting in that condition.[10]

Summary

The adaptation of radioactive tracer techniques has evolved considerably since the cloud chamber and radioactive sodium were used to measure circulation time. We are now able to evaluate objectively aspects of the peripheral circulation, such as regional distribution of blood flow under various physiologic conditions or the blood flow to a specific muscle group, which are otherwise not clinically obtainable by other means. In addition, radioisotopic techniques provide a safe, simple means of quantifying various clinical conditions such as the presence and magnitude of arteriovenous communications or the ability to sustain hyperemic response to injury. Nuclear medicine has provided physiologic, prognostic and diagnostic information previously unobtainable or attainable only with more invasive techniques. In due course, these techniques should become common place in a community hospital and be applied to a patient being evaluated for peripheral arterial disease.

References

1. Lassen, N.A., and Holstein, P.: Use of radioisotopes in assessment of distal blood flow and distal blood pressure in arterial insufficiency. *Surg Clin N Am* **54**:39, 1974.
2. Serjrsen, P.: Epidermal diffusion barrier to ^{133}Xe in man and studies of clearance of ^{133}Xe by sweat. *J Appl Physiol* **24**:211-216, 1968.
3. Siegel, M.E., Giargiana, F.A., Rhodes, B.A., et al.: Effect of reactive hyperemia on the distribution of radioactive microspheres in patients with peripheral vascular disease. *Am J Roentgen* **118**:814-819, 1973.
4. Moss, C.M., Rudavsky, A.Z., and Veith, F.J.: The value of scintiangiography in arterial disease. *Arch Surg* **111**:1235-1242, 1976.
5. Rudavsky, A.Z., Moss, C.M., and Veith, F.J.: Role of isotope angiography in evaluation of arterial injury. Presented at World Federation of Nuclear Medicine and Biology, Washington, D.C., 1978.
6. Meindok, H.: Visualization of arterial and arteriole graft patency by intravenous radionuclide angiography. *Canad Med Assoc J* **106**:1180-1182, 1972.
7. Moss, C.M., Rudavsky, A.Z., and Veith, F.J.: Isotope angiography: Technique, validation and value in assessment of arterial reconstruction. *Ann Surg* **184**:116-121, 1976.
8. Strauss, H.W., Harrison, K., Langan, J.K., et al.: Relation of Thallium-201 to regional myocardial perfusion. *Circulation* **51**:641-645, 1975.
9. Strauss, H.W., Harrison, K., and Pitt, B.: Thallium-201: Noninvasive determination of the regional distribution of cardiac output. *J Nucl Med* **18**: 1167-1170, 1977.
10. Siegel, M.E.: Tl-201: A new approach to peripheral vascular disease. In

Proceedings of the Second Congress of the World Federation of Nuclear Medicine and Biology, 1978.

11. Rhodes, B.A., Greyson, N.D., Siegel, M.E., et al.: The distribution of radioactive microspheres in patients with peripheral vascular disease. *Am J Roentgen* **118**:820, 1973.

12. Siegel, M.E., and Wagner, H.N., Jr.: Radioactive tracers in peripheral vascular disease. *Sem Nucl Med* **6**:253, 1976.

13. Siegel, M.E., Giargiana, F.A., White, R.I., et al.: Peripheral vascular scanning: Correlation with the arteriogram and clinical assessment in the patient with peripheral vascular disease. *Am J Roentgen* **125**:628-633, 1975.

14. Rhodes, B.A., Greyson, N.D., Hamilton, C.R., et al.: Absence of anatomic arteriovenous shunts in Paget's disease of bone. *N Engl J Med* **287**:686-689, 1972.

CHAPTER XX

Mobile Nuclear Medicine Instrumentation

Robert E. Henkin, M.D.

While most radionuclide imaging is done in the department of nuclear medicine, transporting some patients is medically unjustified. This group of patients comprises those individuals whose medical conditions are unstable, who are linked to life-support systems, or in whom the pain and discomfort of transport outweigh the benefit of the nuclear medicine examination. Until recently this patient group could not benefit from nuclear medicine studies.

Beginning in the mid 1970's, gamma cameras designed specifically to image patients at the bedside were marketed by several manufacturers. At the time these devices were introduced, the applications of nuclear medicine to cardiology were in their infancy. It immediately became evident that the needs of the cardiac patient made him particularly well suited to imaging via mobile instrumentation. Shortly after the introduction of mobile gamma cameras, it became evident that computer processing of studies for cardiac patients was not only desirable but highly beneficial. Measurements of left ventricular ejection fraction, wall motion, and cardiac output, as well as results of drug interventions could easily be imaged and quantified using data processing equipment.[1-3] Consequently, data processing equipment was developed to be integrated into the mobile gamma camera or to act as a companion to the gamma camera (Figs. 20-1 and 20-2).

Instrumentation

A 15-inch field of view gamma camera head weighs approximately 2,000 pounds. Although it has wheels so that it can be moved around, its size and space requirements limit its mobility. Well-designed portable

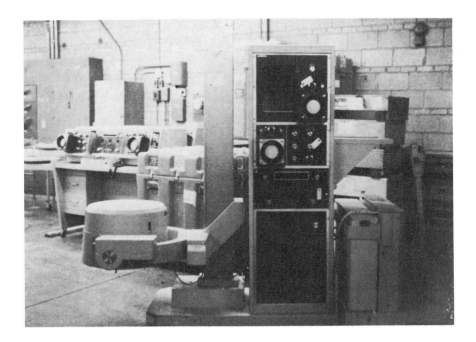

Figure 20-1. An early mobile scintillation camera consisted of a Pho/Gamma HP camera mounted on a hand truck so that it could be moved through the hospital.

scanning equipment must be more than a camera that can be pushed from one location to the other. The camera must be small and maneuverable enough to be moved around life-support equipment. It is desirable, but not essential, that the device be operated by a single individual, since the cost of assigning two technologists as a minimum staff raises the cost of examinations.

Because of these requirements, mobile gamma cameras are generally available in the 10-inch format. At the present, 10-inch gamma cameras have better resolution than their 15-inch counterparts. Therefore, one may expect that the quality of a study from a mobile gamma camera will be at least equal to that of the stationary gamma camera in the Department of Nuclear Medicine. Mobile gamma cameras are smaller and lighter than stationary ones because the amount of shielding is reduced in the mobile cameras. The shielding on mobile gamma cameras is adequate for isotopes up to approximately 200 keV photon energy. Studies using technetium-99m, xenon-133 (80 keV) and iodine-123 labeled products (159 keV) could be done on the mobile devices; however, studies using isotopes such as iodine-131 (364 keV), gallium (93 keV, 184

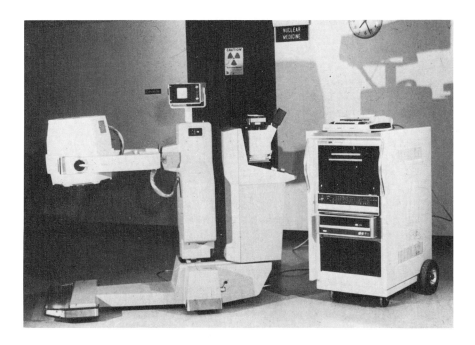

Figure 20-2A. Typical mobile instrumentation available today includes lightweight mobile gamma camera as well as mobile dedicated data processing devices. *A,* Searle LEM and Medical Data Systems RAS.

keV, 300 keV), indium-111 (173 keV, 247 keV) and other high energy isotopes cannot be done on portable cameras.

Nuclear medicine mobile equipment is used primarily for lung scanning, myocardial infarction imaging with phosphates, thallium imaging and first-pass or gated blood pool studies. Other uses of mobile instrumentation involve studies of liver and spleen in patients with traumatic injuries, studies of cerebral death (Fig. 20-3) brain scanning, and renal flow or dynamic studies of major vessels.

Data processing equipment for mobile instrumentation has developed along two lines. The first of these, the integrated approach, incorporates the data processing device into the gamma camera itself. This approach has the advantage of creating a single device to be transported and assuring that the interfacing between the data processor and gamma camera is always correct and on line. The disadvantage of this approach is that it creates a bulkier mobile device which generates more heat in the patient room and occupies more space. A second disadvantage of this method is that one may not be able to purchase the best combination of

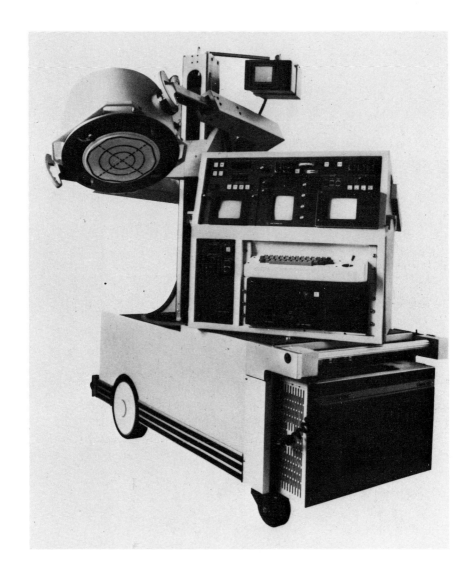

Figure 20-2B.   Ohio Nuclear portable gamma camera.

data processor and gamma camera. The operator must use whichever data processing system is built into the camera system.

We use separate data processing and gamma camera devices. This alternative system has the advantage of allowing the purchaser to purchase the best device for each application. Mobile data processing devices may be acquired directly from data processing companies while the

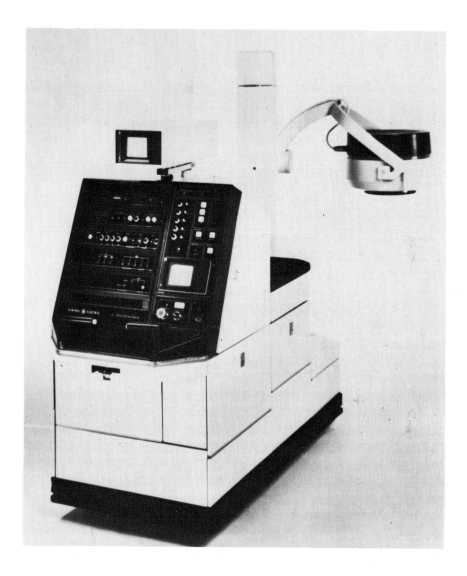

Figure 20-2C. General Electric models of portable gamma cameras have integrated computer systems.

gamma camera may be purchased independently. In general, interfacing is relatively simple. The gamma camera is connected to the computer by x, y, and z cables. The camera must be connected to the computer before an acquisition is begun.

With a component system, the computer may be left outside the patient's room. The cable connects the computer to the camera inside

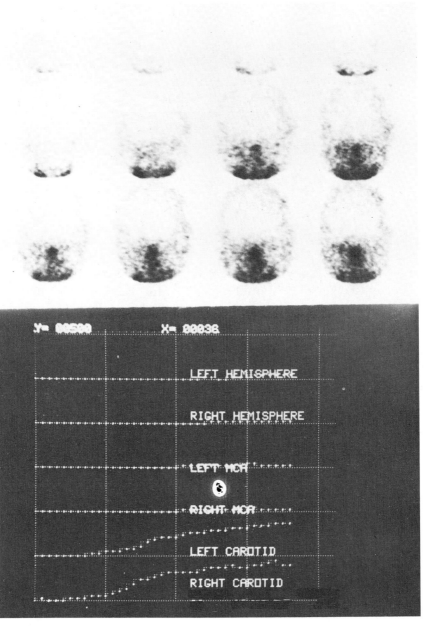

Figure 20-3.   The upper images of a flow study in a patient with suspected cerebral death. No intracranial vasculature or sinuses are demonstrated. The computer-processed curves demonstrate no significant blood flow in the cerebral hemisphere. The findings are consistent with cerebral death. The study was done at the bedside in the intensive care unit.

the patient's room. This system permits greater mobility in cramped quarters and decreases the heat production in the patient's room. A remote control system for the computer is needed at the gamma camera console. In general, this requirement has not proven to be a significant problem. Additionally, this approach permits the tailoring of the computer system. Providing a free-standing additional computer is available for processing, unnecessary displays and data processing options can be eliminated, thus decreasing cost.

Clinical Studies

Thallium Scanning

Current recommendations for imaging with thallium during stress testing suggest that inordinately long intervals between injection and imaging cause thallium to be redistributed. Therefore, if the nuclear medicine facility is not located near the stress testing laboratory, it may be necessary to use mobile instrumentation at the site of stress testing. Gamma cameras may be specially modified for thallium imaging. This modification consists of replacing the standard ½-inch sodium iodide crystal in the gamma camera with a ¼-inch crystal. The ¼-inch crystal produces better resolution at the thallium's low energy levels without degrading resolution at other energy levels. There is however, approximately a 15 percent loss in sensitivity at the energy levels of technetium-99m.

Studies done in our laboratory with the ¼-inch gamma camera crystal have demonstrated superior resolution at thallium's energy levels. Therefore, we have chosen to use ¼-inch crystal mobile gamma cameras for all of our thallium studies. If a patient's images are taken on a ¼-inch crystal camera during stress testing, the images of that patient at rest should be taken on the same equipment. Using a device with less resolution might give the impression that a defect identified on the stress study is reversible, when in truth it has not been resolved because of poorer resolution.

Myocardial Infarction Imaging

The simplest application of the gamma camera is to image patients with myocardial infarctions. In general, this study is easily carried out in the cardiac care unit whether or not the data processing is done there. It is unnecessary to move the patient from his room at a time when transportation is considered hazardous.

Gated Blood Pool Studies

When the gamma camera is coupled with mobile data processing equipment, the technician may conduct gated blood pool imaging at bedside. The determination of left ventricular ejection fraction, wall motion and response to therapeutic interventions, is easily and sequentially measured without ever moving the patient from his room. The condition of patients who are critically ill and on life-support systems may be evaluated sequentially until they are stable enough to be moved for further diagnostic procedures.

This technique offers a reliable means of delivering reproducible data on ejection fraction, segmental wall motion, chamber volumes and cardiac output, adding a dimension never before achieved in the management of critically ill patients. The risk to the patient is insignificant and about the same as that of a brain scan.

Lung Scanning

Transporting patients from the coronary care unit or other special care units to Nuclear Medicine for lung scanning has always created some tension within the Department of Nuclear Medicine, if not among the clinical staff. With the advent of the mobile equipment, excellent perfusion lung scans may be performed quickly at the patient's bedside. Unlike portable x-rays, the quality of the mobile lung scan is equal to that of a scan taken in the nuclear medicine department.

With appropriate amendments to the institution's Nuclear Regulatory Commission license, even mobile ventilation scanning may be carried out at the bedside. The ability to diagnose pulmonary embolic disease in critically ill patients without relocating them is a significant advantage. Follow-up studies may be taken in a similar fashion (Fig. 20-4).

Renal Flow Studies

In patients with decreased urinary output or suspicion of renal arterial lesions, especially in patients who have had renal transplants and who cannot be moved, it is occasionally desirable to be able to obtain information on the flow to the kidneys. Mobile gamma cameras, especially those coupled with data processing devices, may provide excellent information on renal perfusion. Unfortunately, iodine-131 Hippuran studies done with these imaging devices do not provide information on renal

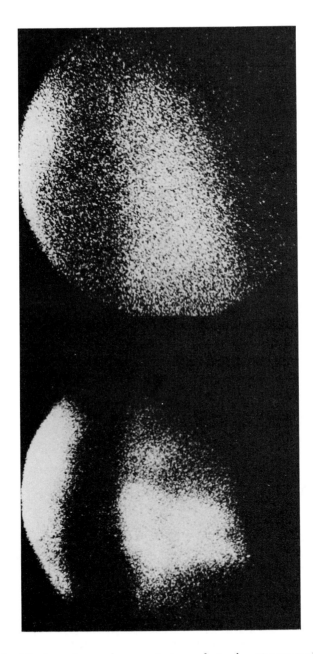

Figure 20-4. The lower image shows posterior perfusion lung image made in the post-operative surgical ICU 24 hours after the patient had surgery. The perfusion scan demonstrated segmental perfusion defects in the right upper lobe. The ventilation in corresponding segments was normal (upper image). The findings were consistent with pulmonary embolic disease. The diagnosis was made in the ICU without moving the patient from bed.

tubular function. Iodine-123 Hippuran is being studied and may prove suitable for use with mobile devices (Fig. 20-5).

Summary

The advent of mobile imaging in nuclear medicine has allowed us to reach out to areas of the hospital where the critically ill patients are housed. These patients who previously could not be studied are now readily accessible.

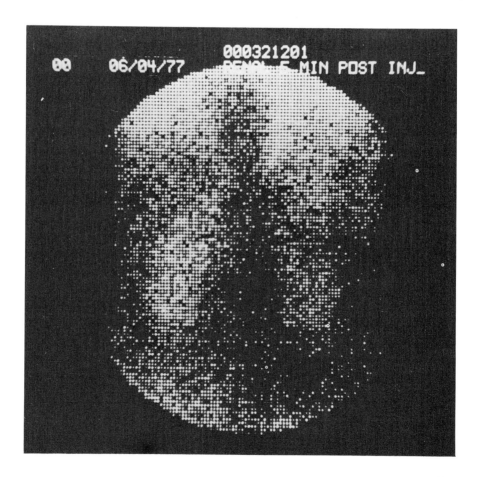

Figure 20-5.   This renal scan of a patient with a dissecting aortic aneurysm demonstrates decreased visualization of the right kidney on the data-processed image. The scan was taken 5 minutes after injection. Arteriography shows that the dissection involves the right renal artery.

The quality of mobile instrumentation is no different from the quality of studies done in the Department of Nuclear Medicine. In general, only a small additional charge is required for a mobile study. All technetium-99m studies may be performed on a mobile basis. In addition, mobile ventilation imaging with xenon-133 is also possible.

In particular, cardiac patients benefit from gated blood pool imaging to quantitate cardiac function at the bedside. Use of mobile imaging equipment in a cardiac care unit is more economically acceptable than the commitment of a stationary imaging device to such a unit. If a stationary imaging device is committed to a cardiac care unit for gated blood pool studies, the device will be significantly underutilized. Indeed, there may be days when no studies at all are required. When mobile equipment is used in such a unit, other studies may be done on the same device in other areas of the hospital.

Stress gated blood pool imaging is best done with mobile instrumentation. In a general hospital it might be difficult to justify a stationary imaging device dedicated to the stress laboratory. However, newer mobile equipment and data processing devices can be brought to the stress laboratory as required for stress gated blood pool imaging. As second generations of mobile gamma cameras become available, it is expected that their flexibility and applications will increase.

References

1. Strauss, H.W., Zaret, B.L., Hurley, P.J., et al.: A scintiphotographic method for measuring left ventricular ejection fraction in man without cardiac catheterization. *Am J Cardiol* **28**:575-580, 1971.
2. Borer, J.S., Bacharach, S.L., Green, M.V., et al.: Real-time radionuclide cineangiography in the noninvasive evaluation of global and regional left ventricular function at rest and during exercise in patients with coronary-artery disease. *N Engl J Med* **296**:839-844, 1977.
3. Bacharach, S.L., Green, M.V., and Borer, J.S.: A real-time system for multi-image gated cardiac studies. *J Nucl Med* **18**:79-84, 1977.
4. Pohost, G.M., Zir, L.M., McKusick, K.A., et al.: Differentiation of transiently ischemic from infarcted myocardium by serial imaging after a single dose of thallium-201. *Circulation* **55**:294-302, 1977.

CHAPTER XXI

Cardiovascular Nuclear Medicine Requirements in a Community Hospital

James H. Thrall, M.D., and Jagmeet S. Soin, M.D.

Cardiovascular disease is the most frequent cause of death among adults today. Because of its prevalence and because it can be treated if properly diagnosed, a great deal of interest has been generated in improving techniques for evaluating cardiovascular disorders. To determine what is needed to offer nuclear cardiological procedures in the community hospital, two things must be considered. First, the functions of the given institution should be determined. For example, requirements for a hospital with a busy coronary care unit but which does no cardiac surgery and little diagnostic stress testing are different from the hospital involved in all of these activities. Second, when the nuclear cardiological studies to be offered have been identified, planners can determine the needed equipment, space, personnel and training. Some of these questions have been reviewed previously by the Intersociety Committee for Heart Disease Resources.[1,2]

Nuclear Cardiology Techniques for Patient Diagnosis and Management

For planning purposes, it is convenient to consider nuclear cardiological procedures in relationship to four broad subdivisions in patient diagnosis and management: (1) medical inpatients, (2) patients undergoing cardiac surgery and (3) patients with congenital heart disease, (4) outpatients with known or suspected coronary artery disease. Each category has distinctly different requirements.

Medical Inpatients—Coronary Care Unit

Coronary Care Units are now a fixture in virtually every hospital either as separate units or in conjunction with other intensive care facilities. Infarct avid imaging, myocardial perfusion imaging and radionuclide ventriculography all have demonstrated utility for diagnosing acute myocardial infarcts but each study also provides other information.

Infarct avid scanning with technetium-99m pyrophosphate may be of particular value in cases where the clinical picture is obscured due to recent infarction, e.g., patients with left bundle branch block and patients with abnormal serum enzymes as a result of operation, congestive heart failure, or trauma. The study also provides information on infarct size and location; and, if baseline studies are done, infarct extension may also be detected.

Thallium-201 myocardial perfusion imaging has the advantage over technetium-99m pyrophosphate of being positive immediately following an acute myocardial infarct. However, the resting thallium scan, as performed on patients with suspected acute myocardial infarctions, cannot distinguish areas of previous infarct with myocardial scarring from acute infarct and/or ischemia without infarction. Nonetheless, thallium-201 may be useful in the early stages following infarction. If performed properly within several hours of infarction, a completely negative study offers fairly good assurance that no infarction has occurred. The study may be useful in triaging coronary care unit admissions.

Radionuclide ventriculography is useful not only for diagnosis but for management of patients in the coronary care unit. Regional wall motion abnormalities are present in a high percentage of patients with acute myocardial infarcts and usually correspond to the acutely damaged myocardial segments. The ability of the heart to pump is readily assessed by calculating ejection fraction and assessing ventricular size. In patients in left ventricular failure, the radionuclide study readily differentiates focal from diffuse disease and provides an objective, direct means of assessing affects of medical therapy. For example, correction of regional wall motion abnormality, improvement in the ejection fraction, and reduction in the end-diastolic volume are favorable findings in response to nitroglycerin therapy. Healing of myocardial infarction can be monitored by taking a series of scans over a period of time. Patients with abnormal ejection fraction have a poorer prognosis than patients whose ventricular function returns to normal following acute myocardial infarcts. This information is of great value to the clinician in counseling patients and may provide a basis for more objectively recommending exercise and work levels during rehabilitation.

Diagnostic Testing for Coronary Artery Disease

Stress testing has become a cornerstone in the evaluation of patients with suspected coronary artery disease. Conventional ECG treadmill or bicycle stress testing is useful but limited by significant numbers of false negative and false positive examinations. Stress thallium imaging and radionuclide ventriculography at rest and during exercise stress have been shown over the past two to three years to be useful additional procedures. Both procedures have high reported sensitivity and in general, their interpretation is not adversely affected by the problems causing false positive or noninterpretable ECG stress tests. Perhaps of more importance, comparative studies have now shown that a combination of ECG stress testing and thallium-201 stress imaging is more sensitive than either procedure alone and similar data are becoming available for stress radionuclide ventriculography.

Cardiac Surgery

Stress thallium imaging and stress radionuclide ventriculography are useful when patients suspected of having coronary artery disease are screened for surgery. The technetium-99m pyrophosphate scan is particularly useful for diagnosing infarctions in patients who have had surgery. In these patients conventional criteria may be useless because of ECG changes and elevated levels of enzymes. Thallium-201 myocardial perfusion imaging with exercise and radionuclide ventriculography with exercise provide objective means of assessing the results of surgery. For example, if a thallium-201 scan shows normal uptake in an area that appeared ischemic before surgery, chances are good that the graft is patent and adequate perfusion has been reestablished. It may also serve as a valuable control for later study if symptoms recur.

Congenital Heart Disease

The major additional procedure which should be available is detection and quantification of both left-to-right and right-to-left shunts. Alderson has discussed this in detail in Chapter 17.

Technical, Logistical and Personnel Requirements for Nuclear Cardiological Procedures

Once a hospital has identified the types of nuclear imaging procedures to be offered, a progam statement can be developed for identifying needed supporting equipment, space and personnel.

Infarct Avid Scanning

Infarct avid scanning can be done on any gamma scintillation camera although current generation high-resolution single crystal cameras are preferred. It is important to note, however, that the intrinsically non-invasive nature of the technetium-99m pyrophosphate scan is compromised if the patient must be moved from the coronary care unit where constant monitoring is available. The best device for infarct avid imaging is therefore a mobile scintillation camera so that the study can be done at the patient's bedside. Alternatively, a satellite nuclear medicine diagnostic facility may be established within or near the coronary care unit (this concept will be discussed in greater detail below).

Thallium-201 Imaging

The thallium-201 perfusion imaging also requires only a gamma scintillation camera. The need for a high quality imaging device is even greater for thallium-201 studies than for technetium-99m pyrophosphate studies because of the low energy level of the thallium-201 isotope. Stress thallium imaging is most efficiently performed in conjunction with stress ECG testing. Laboratories equipped for ECG stress testing, already have the monitoring equipment and emergency supplies needed for the radionuclide stress studies. In equipping a new facility, these additional equipment needs must not be overlooked.

An additional consideration with stress thallium scans is that imaging should begin within five minutes after the tracer is injected. Internal redistribution of thallium begins almost immediately, and therefore, imaging must begin at once if stress-induced perfusion abnormalities are to be well demonstrated. If combined nuclear cardiology or adjacent facilities are not available, the logistics of transferring a patient from the stress ECG lab to the nuclear imaging department must be arranged in advance to avoid delays. Optimally, however, the two laboratories should be located close to each other. In hospitals where both the ECG stress lab and the nuclear medicine clinic are existing facilities, this requirement may be met by using a mobile camera. At both the University of Michigan Medical Center and the Hospitals of the Medical College of Wisconsin this approach has been satisfactory. All thallium stress studies are done during two or three half-days a week. The mobile camera is used more efficiently than if the studies were scheduled randomly and the time constraints are readily met for beginning the imaging immediately after exercise. In the past, computers have not been considered mandatory for thallium imaging. High quality analog images are acceptable and both Polaroid and transmission film formats have been used in various centers. Where computers are available, image processing with background subtraction has been of some value and more recently, computer-assisted diagnostic schemes have been described for comparing rest and redistribution images quantitatively. Initial reports suggest this approach is significantly more sensitive than visual inspection alone. Computer analysis is also more objective and computers should now at least be considered for thallium imaging.

Radionuclide Ventriculography

Equipment necessary for radionuclide ventriculography depends directly on whether the first pass or the gated blood pool approach is used and for the latter, whether several frames are taken or only dual gated end-diastolic and end-systolic images. As discussed in Chapter 13, the simplest approach to radionuclide ventriculography is to use a gamma scintillation camera with an intravascular tracer and an ECG gate to acquire analog images representing end-systole and end-diastole. This procedure has been largely abandoned in favor of the multiple gated format which requires a computer. First transit studies generally require a computer and may or may not require a gate depending on the exact technique.

Exercise radionuclide ventriculography requires an ergometer in addition to the gamma scintillation camera and computer. The ergometer should be accurately calibrated so that reliable records can be made of exercise work loads. As with thallium stress imaging, equipment for continuously monitoring the patient should be available as should a defibrillator and emergency supplies. If the patient exercises in a supine position, a reinforced imaging table is needed. For upright exercise the bicycle ergometer must be modified to allow close and stable positioning of the patient relative to the gamma camera.

The requirement for a computer increased the logistical problems for doing portable radionuclide ventriculography at the bedside. Since bedside examination appears to be a valuable procedure in managing patients with acute myocardial infarcts and patients who have had surgery, considerable care should be given to acquiring the gamma camera/computer system. Three approaches to remote data acquisition have been developed and are currently used. In well-defined situations where installation is not a problem and examinations are done at a limited number of sites, coaxial cables can be used to transmit data from remote locations to a centrally located nuclear medicine computer. At one center, this approach has been used successfully for a gamma camera located over one mile from the computer facility. However, long cables require amplification of the signal, and special attention must be given to adequate shielding to eliminate significant reflectance if several outlets are tied into one cable.

The alternatives to fixed transmission cables are either a separate mobile computer to be used with the mobile scintillation camera or an integrated mobile gamma camera/computer system. Either of these latter approaches provides greater flexibility because nuclear cardiologic studies can be done at any site accessible to the equipment. However, it is strongly recommended that before any equipment is purchased, the size of doorways, hallways, and rooms be checked to insure that the mobile equipment can actually be brought to the patient's bedside for imaging. A useful means of checking compatibility of sizes is to build a full scale cardboard mock-up of the device. Flexibility of camera head position and length of head extension capability must also be considered when positioning the camera over the patient. Experience with both an integrated camera/computer system and separate mobile camera and mobile computer combinations suggests that the integrated systems are far more efficient of time and personnel since only a single device must be moved and no interface cables need be attached. Table 21-1 summarizes equipment needs for the major types of studies.

Administration and Personnel

Since the accessibility of nuclear medicine facilities is a requirement of the Joint Commission on Accreditation of Hospitals, most institutions which are in a position to consider offering nuclear cardiological procedures will have an existing nuclear medicine facility and a physician qualified to use radioactive materials. Nuclear pharmacy support, equipment maintenance, quality control and health physics planning can all be handled in the existing facility. For studies requiring exercise stress or drug intervention, close coordination between the nuclear medicine physician and cardiologist is necessary and, indeed, successful performance of these studies requires an integration of skills from both disciplines.

Skills of registered technologists are sufficient for static imaging. Additional training is usually required to learn proper use of physiologic synchronizers and ergometers. Significant additional training is required when a computer is used. In practice, not every technologist will be able

TABLE 21-1
Equipment For Nuclear Cardiology Procedures

Equipment	Shunt Detection and Quantification	Infarct Avid Scanning	Thallium-201 Myocardial Scanning		Radionuclide Ventriculography			
			Rest	Stress	Dual ED/ES	Gated Multi-Frame	First Pass	Exercise
1. Gamma Camera	X	X	X	X	X	X	X	X
2. Dedicated Nuclear Medicine Computer System	X		O	O		X	X	X
3. ECG Gate					X	X		X
4. Ergometer/Exercise Apparatus				X				X
5. ECG Monitor and Defibrillator				X				X

X = Required
O = Optional

to acquire the new skills needed for computer data acquisition and processing. In addition, the procedures for exercise radionuclide ventriculography are more difficult than those of other nuclear medicine studies and will most likely require additional training of both physician and technologist who must work in close coordination.

It is helpful to assign two technologists to stress testing procedures so that the equipment can be used fully. In the case of thallium-201 stress imaging, one technologist can be scanning the first patient while the second technologist is in the exercise laboratory with the next patient. This technologist injects the radiotracer during maximal stress, helps the cardiology team with post-stress monitoring and can immediately transfer the patient for imaging. For stress radionuclide ventriculography, one technologist oversees the acquisition and analysis of computer data while the second technologist positions the patient, attaches electrodes, injects the radiotracer, takes hard copy records of ECG's at each stress level, positions the gamma camera head and assists the cardiologist with the ergometer.

All personnel working in the stress testing laboratory should be familiar with cardiopulmonary resuscitation techniques and it is worthwhile for nuclear medicine technologists assigned to stress imaging procedures to receive cardiopulmonary resuscitation training.

Space Requirements

Standard nuclear imaging rooms of 250 to 300 square feet are adequate for cardiological studies including stress ventriculography (Fig. 21-1). If a computer is housed in the same room, additional space may be required. Computers require a dust-free environment where temperature and humidity can be controlled. These conditions should have already been provided for the gamma camera but additional capacity may be required. If the computer is housed in a separate room, adequate air conditioning and filtering must be provided. Having the computer in the same room is convenient for data acquisition and allows the technologist to check the adequacy of a study without leaving the patient. However, for analysis and display of completed procedures and for review with referring physicians, a separate computer room should be provided. The imaging area can then be used and new data acquisition will not be disturbed.

Establishment of Specialized Nuclear Cardiology Diagnostic Units

In hospitals with either a patient population large enough to justify a

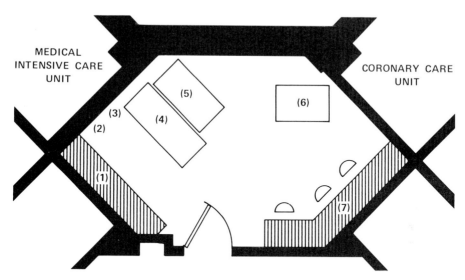

Figure 21-1. A proposed design for nuclear cardiology center. Following is the key to the numbers in the figure: (1) Counter top work area for radiopharmaceutical preparation. Storage cabinets above and below. (2) Wall mounted defibrillator, ECG gate, non-fade oscilloscope and recorder. (3) Oxygen and vacuum outlets at head of imaging table. (4) Reinforced imaging table with floor cleats. (5) Portable gamma camera. (6) Dedicated Nuclear Medicine mini-computer. (7) Desk and counter area for computer terminals and dictating equipment. File drawers below counter.

TABLE 21-2. Nuclear Cardiology Study Unit: Sample Program Planning Statement

---

    I. Function—Performance of Nuclear Cardiology Studies Including:
        -Gathering and analysis of data
        -Record storage (in computer tape and disk form)
        -Practical experience for students and residents

   II. Occupancy
        -Primary—1 patient, 2 technologists, 1 M.D.
        -Secondary—1 student, 2 residents
        -Others—nurse, computer technician

  III. Fixed Equipment
        -Computer 1-46 $\times$ 34 $\times$ 64½
        -Teletype 1-20 $\times$ 20 $\times$ 7
        -Wall Mounted Tape Storage Racks 2
        -Ceiling Mounting Track for track mounted equipment
        -Counter and Shelf for injection supplies
        -Counter or Desk for computer work
        -Shelf or Cabinet for sheets and pillow cases (6 sets per day)
        -Shelf for G.M. Survey Meter

IV. Movable Equipment
-Gamma Camera 56 × 30 × 76.7
-Pedal Mode Ergometer 16W × 36L
-Imaging Table 72 × 30 × 33
-Defibrillator 1-9⅛ × 17⁹⁄₁₆ × 15
-Videotape Recorder 1-23⅜ × 9 × 16½
-Electrocardiograph 1-9⅛ × 26½ × 18
-Emergency Kit 8 × 16 × 10
-Geiger Meuller Survey Meter-12 × 8 × 10
-PLES Resolution Phantom
        57 Co. Flood Source (10" flat disk)
        57 Co. Spot Marker
-Collimator-stored inside camera
-Dry waste receptacle
-Chairs (3)
-Desk (1) or Counter
-File Cabinet
-Gate (Physiological Synchronizer)

V. Utilities and Communications
-Electricity-120 Vac 10A camera
            120 Vac 30A dedicated line for computer
            120 Vac 20A defibrillator
            120 Vac other
-Telephone
-Code blue station to paging
-HVAC-A/C for computer

VI. Special Requirements
-Large door (for camera to pass through)
-Cleats on floor for imaging table
-Shades to provide semi-darkness

VII. Lighting
-Examination Room standard with dimmer
-Light on work surface. For patient's comfort, avoid direct glare over imaging
 table.

VII. Finishes
-Hard floor surface for portable equipment

IX. Other Considerations
-Relocate pneumatic tube station
-Relocate centrex phone console
-Relocate 10E sample refrigerator
-Relocate reception function

Notes:
    (1) All measurements in inches (length × width × height)
    (2) "Other Considerations" are obviously specific to the institution for which this
        statement was developed but are included to emphasize necessity for compre-
        hensive planning to accomodate existing functions displaced by a new activity.

separate dedicated nuclear cardiological unit, or in centers with coronary care and other types of intensive care units clustered in one area of the hospital, it may be feasible and efficient to establish a nuclear medicine satellite either within or close to the intensive care area. There are several special logistical and administrative problems that must be solved in establishing such a diagnostic unit, many of which are the result of being in a location remote from the main department of nuclear medicine.

Radiopharmaceuticals must be transported in a safe manner and a facility must be provided for their temporary storage within the diagnostic unit. After use, syringes and other injection paraphernalia must be returned to the main nuclear medicine pharmacy for disposal. Dosages dispensed from the central radiopharmacy should be recorded so that all radiopharmaceuticals dispensed are recorded in one set of records. Thus errors are reduced. There is a definite burden on the technologist to maintain not only good standards of radiation health, but to comply with all necessary record keeping requirements.

Other logistical problems associated with the remote location include developing film when the unit is not near a darkroom, generating reports and distribution. If outpatients are to be studied, a waiting area is needed and accommodations must be made for scheduling and reception. If the nuclear medicine technologist assists in scheduling and reception, the extra time demands must be considered before determining the number of people assigned to the section.

In planning a nuclear medicine satellite unit it is extremely helpful to develop a program statement. A sample used in establishing a nuclear cardiology diagnostic unit at the University of Michigan Medical Center is provided in Table 21-2. The statement provides information for the hospital architect in determining design specifications and for the hospital administration procuring space and equipment. A comprehensive outline helps insure that no vital piece of equipment is overlooked.

Since most hospitals will be adding these satellite units by remodelling facilities already in use, there will undoubtedly be constraints on size and location. Remodelling necessitates certain compromises but careful architectural design and use of wall mounted and ceiling mounted equipment help make efficient use of available space. Figure 21-1 illustrates a floor plan of a nuclear cardiology diagnostic unit established immediately adjacent to the Medical Intensive and Coronary Care Units at the University of Michigan Medical Center by remodelling a nursing station. The total area is approximately 275 square feet.

In most states, the establishment of any new diagnostic unit will require a Certificate of Need application or similar documentation for review by health care planning agencies. For this purpose as well as for hospital administrative planning, a financial program statement must also be developed to evaluate impact on budget. In addition to direct equipment and commodity costs, indirect costs of reallocating space and possibly establishing a separate call schedule must be included for technologists conducting cardiological procedures. It should also be noted that in preparing financial program statements, incremental costs for performing the various nuclear cardiological procedures are quite different. For example, radiotracer cost for a thallium-201 perfusion scan is on the order of four to six times the cost for radiotracers used in gated blood pool study. Table 21-3 summarizes the relative cost of nuclear cardiology procedures.

Conclusion

Progress in the development of nuclear cardiological studies has been rapid in the past several years. The development and clinical availability of new tracers, imaging instruments and computers have facilitated the transition from almost exclusively research interest to broad clinical applications. Each medical center must determine the specific role for nuclear imaging techniques within the context of services offered at that facility. Guidelines have been presented for aiding decisions in equipment acquisition and facilities planning.

TABLE 21-3
Relative Cost for Nuclear Cardiac Studies Discussed in Arbitrary Units

	Cost Unit
STUDY: Acute Myocardial Infarction	
1. Tc-99m Pyrophosphate Scan	1
2. Tl-201 Myocardial Scan (rest)	1.5
3. Multiple Gated Acquisition (MUGA)	
At Bedside	1.75
STUDY: Myocardial Ischemia	
4. Tl-201 Myocardial Scan (Exercise)	
with Delayed Images	2.5
5. MUGA (Exercise)	2.0
6. MUGA (Rest)	1.25
7. Radionuclide Angiography	1
8. Shunt Detection (Quantitation)	1.5
9. Nuclear Probe Studies	
For Left Ventricular Ejection Fraction	1

References

1. Adelstein, S.J., Jansen, C., and Wagner, H.N., Jr.: Optimal resource guidelines for radioactive tracer studies of the heart and circulation. *Circulation* **52**:A-9/A-22, 1975.
2. Adelstein, S.J.: Organization of cardiovascular nuclear medicine units. *Am J Cardiol* **38**:761-765, 1976.

Index